Pocket Guide to MR Procedures and Metallic Objects: Update 1999

Frank G. Shellock, Ph.D.
Adjunct Clinical Professor of Radiology
University of Southern California
School of Medicine
Los Angeles, California
and Shellock R&D Services, Inc.
Los Angeles, California

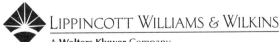

A **Wolters Kluwer** Company
Philadelphia • Baltimore • New York • London
Buenos Aires • Hong Kong • Sydney • Tokyo

Lippincott Williams & Wilkins, 227 East Washington Square,
Philadelphia, Pennsylvania 19106

© 1999 by Lippincott Williams & Wilkins. All rights reserved. This book is
protected by copyright. No part of it may be reproduced, stored in a retrieval
system, or transmitted, in any form or by any means, electronic, mechanical,
photocopying, recording, or otherwise, without the written permission of the
publisher.

Made in the United States of America

Library of Congress Cataloging-in-Publication Data

Shellock, Frank G.
    Pocket guide to MR procedures and metallic objects: update
1999/Frank G. Shellock
    p. cm.
  Includes bibliographical references.
  ISBN 0-781-72345-0
  1. Magnetic resonance imaging—Complications—Handbooks,
manuals, etc. 2. Metals in medicine—Magnetic properties—Handbooks,
manuals, etc. 3. Implants, Artificial—Magnetic properties—Handbooks,
manuals, etc. I. Title.
  [DNLM: 1. Magnetic Resonance Imaging—contraindications—handbooks.
2. Nuclear Magnetic Resonance—handbooks. 3. Metals—handbooks.
4. Implants, Artificial—handbooks. WN 39 S545p 1999]
RC78.7.N83S54 1999
616.07′548—dc20
DNLM/DLC
for Library of Congress   95-42237
                                                                           CIP

    The material contained in this volume was submitted as previously
unpublished material, except in the instances in which credit has been given to
the source from which some of the illustrative material was derived.
    Great care has been taken to maintain the accuracy of the information
contained in the volume. However, neither Lippincott Williams & Wilkins nor
the author can be held responsible for errors or for any consequences arising
from the use of information contained herein.

9 8 7 6 5 4 3 2 1

Disclaimer

The author and publisher of this work accept no legal responsibility for any injury and/or damage to persons or property from any of the methods, products, instructions, or ideas contained herein.

Because of the ongoing research, equipment modifications, and changes in governmental regulations, no suggested product information should be used unless the reader has reviewed and evaluated the information provided with the product.

To Jaana Shellock, a truly extraordinary person,
a gentle soul, and kindred spirit.
Mina rakastan sinua!

To Jaan Cohan, Baby Dumpling, Nala, and Ren.

Contents

Acknowledgments vi

Introduction 1

Information Concerning Implants, Materials, Devices, and
Objects Evaluated for Compatibility with MR Procedures 8

MR Procedures and Patients with Electrically Activated
   Implants and Devices 46

Magnetically Activated Implants and Devices 65

Screening Patients with Metallic Foreign Bodies 68

Screening and Protecting Individuals and Patients From
   "Missile Effect" Injuries 71

Tattoos, Permanent Cosmetics, and Eye Makeup 73

Safety Considerations for the Extremity MR System 76

Future Considerations of Bioimplants, Materials, Devices,
   and Objects 80

Summary 82

References 83

List of Items Tested 95

References 169

Appendix I: Medical Devices Developed for
Interventional MR Procedures 174

Appendix II: Email Address for Frank G. Shellock, Ph.D. .. 192

Acknowledgments

Special thanks to Dr. Emanuel Kanal for his friendship and multiple contributions to the "list."

I am indebted to my brother, Vincent J. Shellock, for the many tedious yet enjoyable hours he devoted to testing bioimplants, devices, and materials with me.

Introduction

Magnetic resonance (MR) procedures may be contraindicated for a patient primarily because of the risks associated with movement or dislodgement of a ferromagnetic biomedical implant, material, device, or object (1–150). Other possible hazards related to the presence of a metallic object include induction of electrical current, excessive heating, and the misinterpretation of an imaging artifact as an abnormality (115).

Induced electrical currents. The potential for MR procedures to injure patients by inducing electrical currents in conductive materials or devices such as gating leads, indwelling catheters with metallic components (e.g., thermodilution catheters), guide wires, disconnected or broken surface coils, certain cervical fixation devices, or improperly used physiologic monitors has been previously reported (13,21, 48,49,55,57,58,112,116,117,119–123,128,132,138,140). Recommendations concerning techniques to protect patients from injuries related to induced current that may develop during an MR procedure, especially those associated with the use of monitoring equipment, have been presented (21,49,55,58,112). Some of these include the following (112,115):

1. Use only devices and monitoring equipment thoroughly tested and determined to be safe for patients during MR procedures.

2. Allow only properly trained individuals to operate devices and monitoring equipment and to be responsible for the patient in the MR environment.

3. Before using the device or equipment, check the integrity of the electrical insulation of the components or accessories of the device including monitoring leads, cables, and wires. Preventive maintenance should be practiced routinely.

4. Remove all electrically conductive material from the bore of the MR system that is not required for the procedure (i.e., unused surface coils, cables, etc.).

5. Keep electrically conductive material that must remain in the bore of the MR system from directly contacting the patient by placing thermal and/or electrical insulation (including air) between the conductive material and the patient.

6. Keep electrically conductive material(s) (e.g., electrocardiographic leads, cables, wires, etc.) that must remain within the bore of the MR system from forming large diameter, conductive loops (remember, the patient's tissue is conductive and, therefore, may be involved in the formation of the conductive loop).

7. Position all cables to prevent "cross points." A cross point is the point where a cable crosses another cable, a cable loops across itself, or a cable touches either the patient or sides of the magnet bore more than once. Note that loops can be closed, U-shaped, or S-shaped.

8. Position all cables and wires so they exit as close as possible to the center of the table of the MR system.

9. Position the patient so there is no direct contact between the patient's skin and the bore of the magnet of the MR system. This may be accomplished by having the patient place his/her arms over his/her head or by using elbow pads or foam padding between the patient's tissue and the magnet bore.

10. Do not position conductive leads, cables, or wires across the area of an external metallic prosthesis or similar device that is in contact with the patient.

11. Devices or equipment that do not appear to be operating properly during the MR procedure should be removed from the patient immediately.

12. If the patient reports feeling warm or hot in association with the use of monitoring equipment or other similar device, discontinue the MR procedure immediately and perform a thorough assessment of the equipment to determine proper functioning.

13. Use only MR system manufacturer-recommended or monitoring equipment manufacturer-recommended electrocardiographic wires, leads, electrodes, and other components and accessories.

14. Follow all instructions for the proper operation of physiologic monitoring or other similar electronic equipment provided by the manufacturer of the device.

Heating. Temperature elevations produced during MR procedures have been studied using *ex vivo* testing techniques to evaluate various metallic implants, materials, devices, and objects of a variety of sizes, shapes, and metallic compositions. In general, these data indicate that only minor temperature changes occur in association with MR procedures involving metallic objects. Therefore, heat generated during an MR procedure involving a patient with a metallic bioimplant does not appear to be a substantial hazard. In addition, there has never been a report of a patient being seriously injured as a result of excessive heat developing in a metallic biomedical implant or device, with the exception of first-, second-, or third-degree burns that occurred in association with induced electrical currents in conductive devices that were not used according to manufacturer's recommendations.

Artifacts. The type and extent of various artifacts caused by metallic implants, materials, and devices have been described and are well-recognized on MR images (65–70,81,82,90–92,95,101, 102,105,110,115–120,124–128,130,131,133,134,142). The distortion of the image by a metallic object is predominantly caused by a disruption of the local magnetic field that perturbs the relationship between position and frequency that is crucial for proper image reconstruction. For this reason, biomedical implants, materials, devices or objects that incorporate magnets can produce artifacts on

MR images that are especially profound because of the accentuated effect of changing the local magnetic field (29,50,58,115–117).

The relative amount of image distortion and artifacts is dependent on the magnetic susceptibility, quantity, shape, orientation, and position of the object in the body as well as the techniques used for imaging (i.e., the specific pulse sequence parameters) and image processing method (i.e., 2D Fourier transform reconstruction, back projection, etc.) (81,82). An artifact caused by the presence of a metallic object in a patient during an MR imaging procedure is seen typically as local or regional distortion of the image and/or as a signal void. In some cases, there may be areas of high signal intensity seen along the edges of the signal void. Notably, the extent, configuration, and characteristics of the artifact are frequently unpredictable.

Nonferromagnetic objects tend to produce artifacts that are less severe than ferromagnetic objects for a given set of MR imaging parameters. Artifacts caused by nonferromagnetic bioimplants result from eddy currents that can be generated in the objects by gradient magnetic fields used for MR imaging that, in turn, disrupt the local magnetic field and distort the image (81,82).

Magnetic field interactions. Numerous studies have assessed the ferromagnetic qualities of various biomedical implants, materials, devices, and objects by measuring deflection forces, attraction, torque or other interactions associated with the static and/or gradient magnetic fields generated by MR systems. With respect to the evaluation of ferromagnetism, these investigations have demonstrated that MR procedures may be performed safely in patients if the metallic object is nonferromagnetic or is ferromagnetic and only minimally attracted (i.e., "weakly ferromagnetic") by the magnetic field in relation to its *in vivo* application or use (i.e., the associated attractive force is insufficient to move or dislodge the object *in situ* or affect its intended function) (115). Accordingly, MR procedures may be performed in patients with bioimplants, materials, devices or objects that have been shown to be nonferromagnetic or "weakly ferromagnetic". [For the sake of discussion, the term "weakly ferromagnetic" refers to metal that may demonstrate some extremely low ferromagnetic qualities using highly sensitive measurements techniques (e.g., vibrating sample magnetometer, superconducting quantum interference device or SQUID magnetometer, etc.) and as such, may not be technically referred to as being "nonferromagnetic". It is further recognized that all metals possess some degree of magnetism, such that no metal is considered to be totally "nonferromagnetic" (125).]

Patients with certain implants or devices that have relatively strong ferromagnetic qualities may be safely scanned using MR because the implants or devices are held in place by sufficient retentive forces that prevent them from being moved or dislodged by the magnetic fields of the MR system. For example, there is an interference screw used for reconstruction of the anterior cruciate ligament that is screwed into the patient's bone, preventing it from being attracted by sufficient force from a 1.5 Tesla (T) magnetic field to move it *in situ* (60). This implant will not heat excessively, although, being ferromagnetic, a rather large signal void is seen on MR imaging (60).

Each bioimplant, material, device, or object (particularly those made from unknown materials) should be evaluated using *ex vivo* techniques before performing an MR procedure in a patient with the specific object (115). By following this procedure, the presence and relative degree of ferromagnetism may be determined so that a competent decision can be made concerning any associated risks due to potential adverse interactions with the magnetic fields of the MR system. Again, because movement or dislodgement of a metallic object in a patient undergoing an MR procedure is the primary mechanism responsible for a possible injury, this aspect of testing is of the utmost importance.

Various factors influence the risk of performing an MR procedure in a patient with a ferromagnetic bioimplant, material, or device including: the strength of the static and gradient magnetic fields, the degree of ferromagnetism of the object, the mass of the object, the geometry of the object, the location and orientation of the object *in situ*, the presence of retentive mechanisms (i.e., fibrotic tissue, bone, sutures, etc.) and the length of time the object has been in place. These factors should be carefully considered before subjecting a patient with a ferromagnetic object to an MR procedure, particularly if it is located in a potentially dangerous area of the body such as near a vital neural, vascular, of soft tissue structure where movement or dislodgement could injure the patient. Furthermore, in certain cases, there is a possibility of changing the operational or functional aspects of the implant, material, or device as a result of exposure to the electromagnetic fields used by the MR systems.

MR systems with very low (0.2 T or less) or very high (2.0 T to 8.0 T) static magnetic fields are currently manufactured and being used for clinical MR applications. Considering that most implants, materials, devices and objects evaluated for magnetic field attraction were assessed at 1.5 T, an appropriate variance or modification of the standard information provided regarding the safety of performing an MR procedure in a patient with a metallic object may exist when an MR system with a lower or higher static magnetic field strength is used. It is probably acceptable to "relax" or adjust the safety recommendations or it may be required to make them more strict, depending on the strength of the MR system's static magnetic field. Performing an MR procedure using a 0.064 T MR system obviously has different risk implications for a patient with a ferromagnetic bioimplant compared with a 8.0 T MR system. Additional discussion of this issue is provided later in this book.

The information contained in this book is a compilation of the current data available on assessment of magnetic field interactions for bioimplants, materials, devices, and objects and primarily based on published reports in the peer-reviewed literature. Additionally, this compilation includes unpublished data that was acquired from *ex vivo* tests of objects that were conducted using the most commonly performed, standardized, and accepted techniques for MR safety. Although every attempt was made to provide comprehensive and accurate information, it should be noted that there are many additional bioimplants, materials, devices, and objects in existence that remain to be evaluated with regard to MR safety. Therefore, to ensure the safety of patients in the MR environment, MR users should follow the guideline whereby MR procedures should only be performed in a patient with a metallic object that has been previously tested and demonstrated to be safe (55, 115).

Information Concerning Implants, Materials, Devices, and Objects Evaluated for Safety with MR Procedures

Although lists of bioimplants, materials, devices, and objects tested for interaction with the magnetic fields of MR systems have been published and updated on several occasions, it is necessary to understand certain aspects of this information and how best to use it for addressing patient safety issues in the MR environment (83). The data presented in any list of this nature represent a specific "snapshot in time" for the period indicated and for the particular bioimplants, materials, devices and objects that have been evaluated using the technique(s) described in the publication (83, 115). Changes in the general information may occur for a variety of reasons. Therefore, a revised version of the "list" is not uncommon and, in fact, necessary.

Manufacturers may change the composition of the bioimplant, material, device, or object without being required to notify or seek new approval from the United States Food and Drug Administration (FDA) as long as the function of the device remains the same (83,85). Therefore, MR facilities may elect to follow guidelines,

Information Concerning Implants and Materials

such as contacting the company that manufactured the device to determine if any alterations in component materials occurred since it was tested previously (83). This is particularly important for those devices that would present a serious hazard to the patient if it was possible that it could be moved or dislodged (e.g., aneurysm clips, otologic implants, etc.) in association with an MR procedure.

Additionally, it is important to note there is now a proliferation of MR systems with static magnetic field strengths that exceed 1.5 T. Very few of the bioimplants, materials, devices, or objects have been assessed to determine the relative amount of attraction to these higher static magnetic fields. Most testing has been conducted using MR systems with static magnetic fields of 1.5 T or lower. Therefore, it is conceivable that there may be an instance where a device that exhibited only "mild" or "slight" ferromagnetism in association with a static magnetic field strength of 1.5 T or lower is now attracted with sufficient force to pose a hazard to a patient or other individual in the MR environment that is associated with an MR system that has a static magnetic field strength of 2.0 T or higher.

Conversely, MR systems designed for use as "dedicated" extremity MR systems have unique features with regards to their magnetic fields. For example, one such extremity MR system (Artoscan, Lunar, Milwaukee, WI and Esaote, Genoa, Italy) has a 0.2 T static magnetic field that has a 5 gauss fringe field contained within approximately 15 inches of isocenter of the device. Because this MR system was designed to image extremities only (e.g., feet, ankles, legs, knees, hands, wrists, elbows, arms), a patient with a metallic object is not subjected to the level of magnetic field forces similar to that produced by an MR system with a conventional design. From a general safety standpoint, the configuration of a low static magnetic field strength, extremity MR system does not present the same degree of potential hazards to a patient with a metallic bioimplant or device. Additional safety information pertaining to the extremity MR system is discussed later in this book.

Aneurysm and Hemostatic Clips

Aneurysm clips. The surgical management of intracranial aneurysms and arteriovenous malformations (AVMs) by the application of aneurysm clips is a well-established procedure. The presence of an aneurysm clip in a patient referred for an MR procedure represents a situation that requires the utmost consideration because of the associated risks. Certain types of intracranial aneurysm clips (e.g., those made from martensitic stainless steels such as 17-7PH or 405 stainless steel) are an absolute contraindication to the use of MR procedures because excessive, magnetically induced forces can displace these clips and cause serious injury or death (5–7,11, 12,21,22,39,46,56,77,78,83,85,115,124,125,127).

By comparison, aneurysm clips classified as "nonferromagnetic" or "weakly ferromagnetic" (e.g., those made from Phynox, Elgiloy, austentitic stainless steels, titanium alloy, or commercially pure titanium) are safe for patients undergoing MR procedures (124,125,127) [For the sake of discussion, the term "weakly ferromagnetic" refers to metal that may demonstrate some extremely low ferromagnetic qualities using highly sensitive measurements techniques (e.g., vibrating sample magnetometer, superconducting quantum interference device or SQUID magnetometer, etc.) and as such, may not be technically referred to as being "nonferromagnetic." It is further recognized all metals possess some degree of magnetism, such that no metal is considered to be totally "nonmagnetic" or "nonferromagnetic."]

It is not uncommon to use MR procedures to evaluate patients with certain types of aneurysm clips. Becker et al. (6), using MR systems that ranged from 0.35 to 0.6 T, studied three patients with nonferromagnetic aneurysm clips (one patient, Yasargil, 316 LVM stainless steel; two patients, Vari-Angle McFadden, MP35N; 316 LVM) and one patient with a ferromagnetic aneurysm clip (Heifetz aneurysm clip, 17-7PH) without incident. Dujovny et al. (11) similarly reported no adverse effects in patients with nonferromagnetic aneurysm clips who have undergone procedures using 1.5 T MR systems.

Of note is that only a single fatality has occurred due to the presence of a ferromagnetic aneurysm clip in a patient preparing to undergo an MR procedure (78). According to the report, the patient involved in this incident complained of a headache at a distance of approximately 1.2 meters from the magnet bore, indicating the translational forces associated with the inhomogeneous component of the magnetic field were responsible for dislodgement of the aneurysm clip (78). This unfortunate incident was the result of erroneous information pertaining to the type of aneurysm clip used in the patient [i.e., the clip was thought to be a nonferromagnetic Yasargil aneurysm clip (Aesculap Inc., South San Francisco, CA) and turned out to be a ferromagnetic Vari-Angle clip (Codman & Shurtleff, Randolf, MA) (78).

There has never been a report of an injury to a patient or individual in the MR environment related to the presence of an aneurysm clip made from a nonferromagnetic or weakly ferromagnetic material. In fact, there have been cases in which patients with ferromagnetic aneurysm clips (based on the extent of the artifact seen during MR imaging or other information) have undergone MR procedures at 1.5 T without any injuries. In these cases, the aneurysm clips were exposed to magnetic-induced translational and torque forces associated with MR systems that had static magnetic fields of up to 1.5 T (personal communications, D. Kroker, 1995 and E. Kanal, 1996) (6). Although these cases do not prove or suggest safety, they demonstrate the difficulty of predicting the outcome for patients with ferromagnetic aneurysm clips that undergo MR procedures.

Unfortunately, there is much controversy and confusion regarding the amount of ferromagnetism that needs to be present in an aneurysm clip to constitute a hazard for a patient in the MR environment. Consequently, this issue has not only created problems for MR healthcare workers but for manufacturers of aneurysm clips, as well. For example, MR users performing test procedures on aneurysm clips similar to that described in the report by Kanal et al. (106), presumably identified the presence of magnetic field interaction and returned several clips made from Phynox to the manufacturer (personal communication, Aesculap, Inc., South San Francisco, CA, 1997).

However, the testing method used by Kanal et al. (106) was admittedly crude and developed to primarily obtain rapid, qualitative screening data for large numbers of aneurysm clips to determine if quantitative data were worth pursuing. Furthermore, this test technique may be problematic and yield spurious results, especially if the aneurysm clips have a shape or configuration that is somewhat "unstable" (unpublished observations, F.G. Shellock, 1997). For example, aneurysm clips with blades that are bayonet, curved, or angled shapes are less stable on a piece of plate glass [i.e., using the testing method described by Kanal et al. (106)] when placed in certain orientations compared with aneurysm clips with blades that have a straight-shape.

A variety of more sophisticated testing techniques have been developed and utilized over the years to evaluate the relative amount of ferromagnetism present for bioimplants and devices prior to allowing patients with these objects to enter the MR environment. The "deflection angle test," originally described by New et al. (39), has been indicated for the specific evaluation of aneurysm clips (draft document entitled, Guidance for Testing MR Interaction with Aneurysm Clips, U.S. Department of Health and Human Services, Food and Drug Administration, Center for Devices and Radiological Health, 1996). The Food and Drug Administration suggests that an evaluation of torque be performed, as well. Procedures such as the deflection angle test and some form of evaluation of torque force utilized to determine the relative amount of ferromagnetism for an aneurysm clip are the most appropriate means of determining which specific clip may present a hazard to a patient or individual in the MR environment.

The deflection angle test is considered to be a useful, reliable, and reproducible test and has been utilized for over 13 years to assess magnetic-induced translational forces for many metallic objects. In 1994, a standard issued from the American Society for Testing and Materials (ASTM) for the requirements and disclosure of aneurysm clips indicated the deflection angle test should be used to specifically evaluate aneurysm clips. Of note is that this document was intended for use by manufacturers, users, engineers, government agencies, and designers of aneurysm clips to provide uniformity in reporting performance characteristics and test methodology.

The ASTM report states that the operational definition of a nonferromagnetic aneurysm clip is met only if the clip passes the following test: "The clip is suspended at the end of a string and held stationary in the vertical direction (that is, perpendicular to the ground) while it is placed in position at the portal of the imaging magnet. Following release of the clip, the deflection of the string from the vertical is then observed. The magnetic force is less than the gravitational force (that is, the clip's weight) if the deflection of the string with respect to the vertical is less than 45 degrees. The clip is then judged to be nonferromagnetic and suitable for implantation."

According to the ASTM, the deflection angle test as described above must be conducted such that the procedure is performed on a "finished" aneurysm clip using a 1.5 T MR system, at the point where the highest spatial gradient field exists for that specific MR system. Although not specified by the ASTM, for most MR systems with a conventional design, the highest spatial gradient is likely to exist somewhere between 30 and 45 cm inside of the bore of the magnet. Therefore, it is at this position the deflection angle test should be conducted. Additionally, it is recommended that a specific length (e.g., 30 cm in length) of 4.0 silk or similar material be used for the test procedure.

The deflection angle test would basically allow aneurysm clips made from weakly ferromagnetic materials to be used in patients undergoing MR procedures (i.e., those aneurysm clips that display deflection angles of between 1 and 44 degrees). Other testing methods, particularly if they are more subjective or insensitive, will not yield the type of information required to adequately determine if an aneurysm clip will present a risk to a patient in the MR environment.

An example of a test that may be performed to qualitatively determine the presence of magnetic field-induced torque for an aneurysm clip is the "Petri dish test." This procedure involves the use of a plastic Petri dish with a millimeter etching on the bottom (alternatively, any material with a flat "slick" or relatively frictionless surface could be used to perform this test). Each aneurysm clip should be placed in the dish in an orientation that is perpendicular to the static magnetic field (preferably a 1.5 T MR system should be used for this evaluation). The Petri dish with the aneurysm clip is then positioned in the center of the MR system, where the effect of torque force from the static magnetic field is known to be the greatest. The aneurysm clip should be directly observed for any type of possible movement with respect to alignment or rotation to the magnetic field. The observation process is facilitated by being inside of the bore of the magnet during the test procedure. The Petri dish with the aneurysm clip should then be brought out of the bore of the magnet, the aneurysm clip should be moved 45 degrees relative to its previous position, re-inserted into the center of the magnet, and again, observed for alignment or rotation. This process should be repeated in order to encompass a full 360-degrees rotation of positions.

In view of the current, knowledge pertaining to aneurysm clips, the following guidelines are recommended for careful consideration prior to performing an MR procedure in a patient with an aneurysm clip or before allowing any other individual with an aneurysm clip into the MR environment:

1. Specific information (i.e., manufacturer, type or model, material, lot and serial numbers) about the aneurysm clip must be known, especially with respect to the material used to make the aneurysm clip, so that only patients or individuals with nonferromagnetic or weakly ferromagnetic clips are allowed into the MR environment. This information is provided in the labeling of every aneurysm clip by the

Information Concerning Implants and Materials

manufacturer. The implanting surgeon is responsible for properly communicating this information in the patient's records.

2. An aneurysm clip in its original package and made from Phynox, Elgiloy, MP35N, titanium alloy, commercially pure titanium or other material known to be nonferromagnetic or weakly ferromagnetic does not need to be evaluated for ferromagnetism. Aneurysm clips made from nonferrromagnetic or weakly ferromagnetic materials in original packages do not require testing of ferromagnetism because the manufacturers ensure the pertinent MR safety aspects of these clips and, therefore, are held responsible for the accuracy of the labeling.

3. If the aneurysm clip is not in its original package or properly labeled, it should undergo testing for magnetic field interactions.

4. Testing for magnetic field interactions should first involve a procedure like the Petri dish test (i.e., for one or a few aneurysm clips) or the procedure described by Kanal et al. (106) (i.e., for screening large numbers of aneurysm clips). If a positive test result is noted using one of these test techniques, then the deflection angle test should be conducted following the guidelines of the ASTM.

5. The radiologist and implanting surgeon should be responsible for evaluating the available information pertaining to the aneurysm clip, verifying its accuracy, obtaining written documentation and deciding to perform the MR procedure after considering the risk vs. benefit aspects for a given patient.

Effects of Long-Term Multiple Exposures to the MR System. Aneurysm clip testing procedures that have been recommended over the past few years would result in the potential for reintroduction of aneurysm clips into strong MR system-related magnetic fields several times prior to ultimate patient implantation (129). Furthermore, there are patients with implanted aneurysm clips that previously tested as "MR compatible" but whom have since undergone repeated exposure to follow-up MR examinations and the concommitant exposure to the strong magnetic fields of these systems.

A concern that recently emerged is that there are potential alterations in the magnetic properties of pre- or post-implanted aneurysm clips resulting from long-term or multiple exposures to strong magnetic fields. Theoretically, long-term or multiple exposures to strong magnetic fields (such as those associated with MR imaging systems) may grossly "magnetize" aneurysm clips, even if they are made from nonferromagnetic or weakly ferromagnetic materials. This scenario would present a significant hazard to an individual in the MR environment. Therefore, an investigation was conducted to study intracranial aneurysm clips *in vitro* prior to and following long-term and multiple exposures to the magnetic fields associated with a 1.5 Tesla MR system (129). This was done to quantify possible alterations in the magnetic properties of the aneurysm clips (129).

Aneurysm clips made from Elgiloy, Phynox, titanium alloy, commercially pure titanium, and austenitic stainless steel were tested in association with long-term and multiple exposures to the strong magnetic fields associated with 1.5 Tesla MR systems (129). The findings of this investigation indicated a lack of response to the various magnetic field exposure conditions used, such that long-term and/or multiple exposures to diagnostic MR examinations or of *in vitro* clips to MR systems for testing purposes should not result in clinically significant changes in their magnetic properties or assessments of their MRI safety (129).

Additional information on performing MR procedures in patients with aneurysm clips is provided in the section titled *Safety Considerations for the Extremity MR System.*

Artifacts Associated with Aneurysm Clips. An additional problem related to aneurysm clips is that artifacts produced by these metallic implants may substantially detract from the diagnostic aspects of MR procedures. It is frequently necessary to evaluate the brain or cerebral vasculature of patients with aneurysm clips using MR imaging or MR angiography. For example, to reduce morbidity and mortality after subarachnoid hemorrhage, it is imperative to assess the results of the surgical treatment of cerebral aneurysms.

The extent of the artifact produced by a given aneurysm clip will have a direct effect on the diagnostic aspects of MR procedures (127). Therefore, an investigation was conducted to characterize the artifacts associated with aneurysm clips made from nonferromagnetic or weakly ferromagnetic materials. Five different aneurysm clips made from five different materials were evaluated in this investigation, as follows:

(1) Yasargil, Phynox (Aesculap, Inc., South San Francisco, CA),
(2) Yasargil, titanium alloy (Aesculap, Inc., South San Francisco, CA),
(3) Sugita, Elgiloy (Mizuho American, Inc., Beverly, MA),
(4) Spetzler Titanium Aneurysm Clip, commercially pure titanium (Elekta Instruments, Inc., Atlanta, GA), and
(5) Perneczky, cobalt alloy (Zepplin Chirurgishe Instrumente, Pullach, Germany).

These aneurysm clips were selected for testing because they are made from nonferromagnetic or weakly ferromagnetic materials and represent the most frequently used aneurysm clips and the latest versions of aneurysm clips that are commercially-available in the United States. Furthermore, these aneurysm clips have been previously reported to be safe for patients in the MR environment and, as such, are often found in patients referred for MR procedures.

The MRI artifact testing revealed the size of the signal voids were directly related to the type of material used to make the particular clip (127). Arranged in increasing order of artifact size, the materials responsible for the artifacts associated with the aneurysm clips were, as follows: Elgiloy (Sugita), cobalt alloy (Perneczky), Phynox (Yasargil), titanium alloy (Yasargil), and commercially pure titanium (Spetzler). These study results have implications when one considers the various critical factors responsible for the decision to use a particular type of aneurysm clip (e.g., size, shape, closing force, biocompatibility, corrosion resistance, material-related effects on diagnostic imaging examinations, etc.) (127). An aneurysm clip that causes a relatively large artifact is less desireable because it can reduce the diagnostic power of MR imaging, or because the area of interest is in the immediate location of where the aneurysm clip was placed (127). Fortunately, manufacturers have developed aneurysm clips made from materials (e.g., commercially pure titanium and titanium alloy) that minimize such artifacts.

Hemostatic clips. To date, none of the various hemostatic vascular clips that have been evaluated were attracted by static magnetic fields up to 1.5 T (46,47,56,62). These hemostatic clips are made from nonferromagnetic materials such as tantalum and nonferromagnetic forms of stainless steel. Therefore, patients that have any of the hemostatic vascular clips listed in the Table are not at risk for injury during MR procedures. There has never been a report of an injury to a patient in association with the presence of a hemostatic vascular clip in the MR environment. Notably, patients with nonferromagnetic hemostatic clips may undergo MR procedures immediately after these clips are placed surgically.

Biopsy Needles, Markers, and Devices

MR imaging has been used to guide tissue biopsy and apply markers with encouraging results. The performance of these specialized procedures requires tools that are compatible with MR systems. Many commercially available biopsy needles, markers, and devices (i.e., guide wires, stylets, marking wires, marking clips, biopsy guns, etc.) have been evaluated with respect to compatibility with MR procedures,

Information Concerning Implants and Materials

not only to determine ferromagnetic qualities but also to characterize imaging artifacts (100,101,113,114). The results indicate most commercially available biopsy needles, markers, devices are not useful for MR-guided biopsy procedures due to the presence of excessive ferromagnetism and the associated imaging artifacts that limit or obscure the area of interest.

For many of the commercially available devices, studies reported the presence of ferromagnetic biopsy needles and lesion marking wires in a tissue phantom used for testing produced such substantial artifacts they would not be useful for MR-guided procedures (100,101). Needles or devices containing any type of ferromagnetic material tend to have too much associated magnetic susceptibility to allow effective use for MR-guided procedures. Fortunately, several needles, markers, and devices have been constructed out of nonferromagnetic materials specifically for use in MR-guided procedures (100,101,113,114). Of note is that certain nonferromagnetic materials, such as titanium, do not appear to have the same constructual integrity properties, which should be carefully considered when selecting an MR-compatible biopsy needle for an MR-guided procedure. For example, Faber et al. (114) reported titanium alloy needles (Somatex, Germany) were weaker and bent more easily during insertion compared to the Inconell (Cook, Germany) or high nickel alloy (E-Z-Em, Westbury, NY) biopsy needles.

Most of the biopsy guns tested for attraction to the static magnetic fields of MR systems were found to be ferromagnetic. Although they are not used in the immediate area of the specific tissue that is to be sampled, the artifact associated with these devices may affect the resulting image during an MR-guided biopsy procedure. Therefore, the presence of ferromagnetism is likely to preclude the optimal use of most biopsy guns in the MR environment. Currently, there is at least one commercially available biopsy gun developed specifically for use in MR-guided procedures that does not have ferromagnetic components (101).

A metallic marking clip, the Micromark, made from 316L stainless steel by Biopsys Medical (Irvine, CA), has been developed for percutaneous placement after stereotactic breast biopsy. The placement of a marking clip is of obvious use, especially in cases where mammographic findings are not apparent or visible (130). The use of a marking clip enables the accurate localization of the surgical excision site and is a useful surrogate target, even when the entire lesion is removed and there is a subsequent need for wire localization prior to surgery. A current limitation of MR-guided needle localization procedures is the inability to document lesion retrieval because it is not possible to perform contrast enhancement of the resected specimen. A Micromark clip placed during MR-guided biopsy or localization can permit radiography to be performed on the surgical specimen to confirm retrieval of the clip and, thus, document retrieval of the lesion (130).

Tests conducted to assess magnetic field interaction, heating, and artifacts indicated the presence of the Micromark clip presents no risk to a patient undergoing an MR procedure using an MR system with a static magnetic field of 1.5 T or less (130). Unfortunately the probe used with the Micromark is strongly attracted by a 1.5 T MR system, preventing its use in this specific MR environment (130). However, the marking clip could be placed outside of the influence of the magnetic field after placement of an MR-compatible introducer.

Breast Tissue Expanders and Implants

Adjustable breast tissue expanders and mammary implants are utilized for breast reconstruction following mastectomy, for the correction of breast and chest-wall deformities and underdevelopment, for tissue defect procedures, and for cosmetic augmentation. These devices are equipped with either an integral injection site or a remote injection dome that is utilized to accept a needle for placement of saline for expansion of the prosthesis intraoperatively and/or postoperatively.

The Becker and the Siltex prostheses are additionally equipped with a choice of a standard injection dome or a micro injection dome. The Radovan expander is indicated for temporary implantation only (101). The injection ports contain 316L stainless steel to guard against piercing the injection port by the needle. There are two different breast tissue expanders constructed with magnetic ports to allow for a more accurate detection of the injection site. These devices are substantially attracted to the static magnetic field of MR systems and, therefore, may be uncomfortable or injurious to a patient undergoing an MR procedure (29).

The relative amount of image distortion caused by the metallic components of these devices should not greatly affect the diagnostic quality of an MR examination, unless the imaging area of interest is at the same location as the metallic portion of the breast tissue expander (101). For example, there may be a situation during which a patient is referred for MR imaging for the determination of breast cancer or a breast implant rupture such that the presence of the metallic artifact could obscure the precise location of the abnormality. In view of this possibility, it is recommended that patients be identified with breast tissue expanders that have metallic components so that the individual interpreting the MR images is aware of the potential problems related to the generation of artifacts. Breast tissue expanders with magnetic ports produce relatively large artifacts on MR images (101).

Cardiovascular Catheters and Accessories

Cardiovascular catheters and accessories are indicated for use in the assessment and management of critically ill or high risk patients including those with acute heart failure, cardiogenic shock, severe hypovolemia, complex circulatory abnormalities, acute respiratory distress syndrome, pulmonary hypertension, certain types of arrhythmias and other various medical emergencies. In these cases, cardiovascular catheters are used to measure intravascular pressures, intracardiac pressures, cardiac output, and oxyhemoglobin saturation. Secondary indications include venous blood sampling and therapeutic infusion of solutions or medications. In addition, some cardiovascular catheters are designed for temporary cardiac pacing and intra-atrial or intraventricular electrocardiographic monitoring.

Because patients with cardiovascular catheters and associated accessories may require evaluation using MR procedures, or because these devices may be considered for use during MR-guided procedures, it is imperative a thorough *ex vivo* assessment be conducted for these devices to ascertain the potential risks of their use in the MR environment. For example, MR imaging, angiography, and spectroscopy procedures may play an important role in the diagnostic evaluation of these patients. Furthermore, the performance of certain MR-guided interventional procedures may require the utilization of cardiovascular catheters and accessories to monitor patients during biopsies, interventions, or treatments.

Notably, there is at least one report of a cardiovascular catheter that melted in a patient undergoing MR imaging (13). Obviously, there are realistic concerns pertaining to the use of similar devices during MR examinations. Therefore, an investigation was conducted using *ex vivo* testing techniques to evaluate cardiovascular catheters and accessories with regard to magnetic field attraction, heating, and artifacts associated with MR imaging (128).

A total of fifteen different cardiovascular catheters and accessories (Abbott Laboratories, Morgan Hill, CA) were selected for evaluation because they represent a wide-variety of the styles and types of devices commonly used in the critical care setting (i.e., the basic structures of these devices are comparble to those made by other manufacturers) (128). Of these devices, the 3-Lumen CVP Catheter, CVP-PVC Catheter (used for central venous pressure monitoring, administration of fluids, and venous blood sampling; polyurethane and polyvinyl chloride, respectively), Thermoset-Iced, and Thermoset-Room (used as accessories for determination of cardiac output using the thermodilution method; plastic), and Safe-set with In-Line Reservoir (used for in-line blood sampling; plastic) were determined to have no metallic components (Personal communications, Ann McGibbon, Abbott Laboratories, 1997) (128). Therefore, these devices were deemed safe for patients undergoing MR procedures and were not included in the overall *ex vivo* tests for MR safety. The remaining ten devices were evaluated for the presence of potential problems in the MR environment (128).

Excessive heating of bioimplants or devices made from conductive materials has been reported to be a hazard for patients who undergo MR procedures (13,115). This is particularly a problem for devices in the form of a loop or coil because current can be induced in this shape during operation of the MR system, to the extent that a first, second or third-degree burn can be produced. The additional physical factors responsible for this hazard have not been identified or well-characterized (e.g., the imaging parameters, specific gradient field effects, size of the loop associated with excessive heating, etc.). For this reason, the previously published study examining cardiovascular catheters and accessories did not attempt to investigate the effect of various "coiled" catheter shapes on the development of substantial heating during an MR procedure. There are many additional factors in addition to the shape of the catheter with a conductive component that can also influence the amount of heating that occurs during and MR procedure (115).

Although a thermodilution Swan-Ganz catheter (specific manufacturer unknown) is constructed of nonferromagnetic materials that includes a conductive wire, a report indicated a portion of this catheter outside the patient melted during MR imaging (13). It was postulated the high-frequency electromagnetic fields generated by the MR system caused eddy current-induced heating of either the wires within the thermodilution catheter or the radiopaque material used in the construction of the catheter (13). This incident suggests patients with this catheter, or a similar device that has conductive wires or other component parts, could be potentially injured during an MR procedure.

Furthermore, heating the wire or lead of a temporary pacemaker (e.g., the RV Pacing Lead) is at least a theoretical concern for any similar wire in the bore of an MR system (115). Cardiac pacemaker leads are typically intravascular for most of their length, and heat transfer and dissipation from the leads into the blood may prevent dangerous levels of lead heating to be reached or maintained for the intravascular segments of pacemaker leads. However, for certain segments of these leads it is at least theoretically possible that sufficient power deposition or heating may be induced within these leads to result in local tissue injury or burn during an MR procedure (115). A recent *ex vivo* study conducted by Achenbach et al. (132) substantiates this contention. Temperature increases of up to 63.1°C were recorded at the tips of pacemaker electrodes during MR imaging performed in phantoms

Because of the deleterious and unpredictable effects, patients referred for MR procedures with cardiovascular catheters and accessories that have internally or externally-positioned conductive wires or similar components should not undergo MR procedures because of the possible associated risks (115,128). Further support of this recommendation is based on the fact that inappropriate use of monitoring devices during MR procedures is often the cause of patient injuries (115). For example, burns have primarily resulted in the MR environment in association with the use of devices that utilize a conductive wire interface to the patient (115).

The cardiovascular catheters and accessories that have been evaluated contained metallic materials that are good electrical conductors which, in turn, could potentially present a hazard for a patient undergoing an MR procedure (128). Therefore, in general, cardiovascular catheters and accessories with conductive metallic components should not be present in patients undergoing MR procedures. Additionally, catheters and accessories from various manufacturers made from a similar design as the devices that were previously tested (i.e., with conductive wire components, etc.) are also likely to present problems to patients in the MR environment (128).

Carotid Artery Vascular Clamps

Each of the different carotid artery vascular clamps tested for ferromagnetism displayed attraction to a 1.5 T static magnetic field (68). However, only the Poppen-Blaylock carotid artery vascular clamp was felt to be contraindicated for patients undergoing MR procedures due to the existence of substantial ferromagnetism (68). The other carotid artery clamps were considered to be safe for patients exposed to the magnetic fields of MR systems because they were only "weakly" ferromagnetic (68). With the exception of the Poppen-Blaylock clamp, patients with metallic carotid artery vascular clamps have been imaged by MR systems with static magnetic fields ranging up to 1.5 T without experiencing any discomfort or neurologic sequelae (68).

Dental Implants, Devices, and Materials

Many of the dental implants, devices, materials, and objects evaluated for ferromagnetic qualities exhibited measurable deflection forces, but only the ones that have a magnetically activated component present a potential problem for patients during MR procedures (see subsequent section, *Magnetically Activated Implants and Devices*) (46,47,56,62). The other dental implants, devices and materials are held in place with sufficient counter-forces to prevent them from causing problems for patients by being moved or dislodged by magnetic fields of MR systems.

ECG Electrodes

A patient should be monitored if there is the potential for a change of physiologic status during the MRI procedure. With the advent of newer types of MRI applications, such as MRI-guided therapy, there is also an increased need to monitor patients in these MRI settings. Studies that need to record the electrocardiogram (ECG) for the purpose of gating also require the proper acquisition of the appropriate physiologic signal for accurate and timely representation of the desired MR images. The use of MRI safe ECG electrodes is strongly recommended to ensure patient safety and proper recording of the electrocardiogram in the MRI environment. Accordingly, ECG electrodes have been specially developed for use during MRI procedures to protect the patient from these potentially hazardous conditions and produce minimal MRI-related artifacts. The "List of Items Tested" provides a compilation of ECG electrodes evaluated for MRI safety.

Foley Catheters With Temperature Sensors

Certain Foley Catheters have temperature sensors to permit recording the temperature of the urine in the bladder, which is a

Information Concerning Implants and Materials

sensitive means of determining "deep" body or core temperature. This type of Foley Catheter typically has a thermistor or thermocouple located on or near the tip of the device and a wire that runs the length of the catheter to a connector that plugs into a temperature monitor. Note, a Foley Catheter with a temperature sensor should never be connected to the temperature monitor during the MR procedure because this equipment is not compatible or safe in the MR environment.

Several of the Foley Catheters with temperature sensors have been evaluated for safety in the MR environment by determining magnetic field interactions, artifacts, and heating (see "List of Items Tested"). In general, the findings of this assessment indicate it would be safe to perform MR procedures on patients using tested Foley Catheters with temperature sensors, when specific recommendations are followed. Similar to any device with a wire component, the position of the wire has an important effect on the amount of heating that develops during an MR procedure. Accordingly, the Foley catheter with a temperature sensor must be positioned in a straight configuration without any loop(s) to prevent possible excessive heating associated with an MR procedure. Furthermore, only conventional pulse sequences should be used (e.g., no echo planar techniques, magnetization transfer contrast, etc.) while imaging with an MR system with a static magnetic field of 1.5 T or less. Additional recommendations include, the following:

(1) If the Foley Catheter with a temperature sensor has a removable catheter connector cable, it should be disconnected prior to the MR procedure.

(2) Remove all electrically conductive material from the bore of the MR system that is not required for the procedure (i.e., unused surface coils, cables, etc.).

(3) Keep electrically conductive material that must remain in the bore of the MR system from directly contacting the patient by placing thermal and/or electrical insulation (including air) between the conductive material and the patient.

(4) Position the Foley Catheter with a temperature sensor in a straight configuration to prevent cross points and conductive loops.

(5) MR imaging should be performed using MR systems with static magnetic fields of 1.5 T or less. Pulse sequences, techniques (e.g., echo planar techniques) or conditions that produce exposures to high levels of RF energy (i.e., exceeding a whole body averaged specific absorption rate of 1.0 W/kg) or exposure to gradient fields that exceed 20-T/second, or any other unconventional MR technique should be avoided.

(6) If the patient reports feeling warm or hot in association with the presence of the Foley Catheter with a temperature sensor, discontinue the MR procedure immediately.

Halo Vests and Cervical Fixation Devices

Halo vests or cervical fixation devices may be constructed from either ferromagnetic, nonferromagnetic, or a combination of metallic components and other materials (4,8,51,102,115,138–140). Although some commercially available halo vests or cervical fixation devices are composed entirely of nonferromagnetic materials, there is a theoretical hazard of inducing electrical current in the ring portion of any halo device made from conductive materials according to Faraday's law of electromagnetic induction (51). Additionally, there is a potential for the patient's tissue to be involved in part of this current loop, so that there would be the possibility of a burn or electrical injury to the patient. The induced current within such a ring or conductive loop is of additional concern because of eddy current induction and potential image degradation effects (138–140). Artifacts associated with the production of eddy currents during MR imaging may be substantially reduced by adjusting the phase encoding direction of the pulse sequences so that it is parallel to the axis of the halo vest (139).

At present, there are no reports of injuries associated with MR procedures performed in patients with halo vests or cervical fixation devices. However, one incident of "electrical arcing" without injury was reported in the 1988 Society for Magnetic Resonance Imaging Safety Survey (Phase I Study; Kanal E, personal communication, 1988). Because of safety and image quality issues, MR procedures should only be performed on patients with specially designed halo vests or cervical fixation devices made from nonferromagnetic and nonconductive materials that have little or no interaction with the electromagnetic fields generated by MR systems (115).

Recently, there have been anecdotal reports of patients with halo vests or cervical fixation devices experiencing sensations of heat during MR imaging procedures. This has also been presumed to be a problem for certain stereotactic headframes used in the MR environment. However, experiments using MR safety test methods demonstrated that there is no heating for at least one such device indicated in the section "List of Items Tested" (unpublished observations, F.G. Shellock, 1996).

A study was conducted to assess the effects of heating halo vests and cervical fixation devices during MR imaging. Testing with a 1.5 T MR system and various pulse sequences used to image the cervical spine the data indicates substantial heating was not detected. Of interest is there appeared to be subtle motions of the halo ring associated with the use of a magnetization transfer contrast (MTC) pulse sequence, as shown by recordings obtained using a motion sensitive, laser-Doppler flow monitor (102). Apparently, the specific imaging parameters used for the MTC pulse sequence produced sufficient vibration of the halo ring to create the sensation of heating. These rapid vibrations may have been felt by the subject and interpreted as a "heating" sensation. This is likely to occur when the frequency and/or amount of vibration is at a certain level that stimulates nerve receptors located in the subcutaneous region that detect sensations of pain and temperature changes.

The aforementioned is merely a hypothesis based on the available experimental data and requires further investigation to substantiate this theory. However, additional support to this premise comes from a report by Hartwell and Shellock (138). In this case, a halo ring and vest (removed from a patient who complained of severe "burning" in a front skull pin during MR imaging) was evaluated for heating or other potential problems associated with MR imaging by the neurosurgeon who applied the device. The halo ring and vest were connected similar to the manner it was used on the patient and a fluid-filled Plexiglas phantom was placed within the vest. The device was then placed within a 1.5 T MR system and MR imaging was performed using the same parameters that were associated with the "burning" sensation experienced by the patient. The neurosurgeon remained within the MR system to visually observe and touch the cervical fixation device during the MR procedure. No perceivable temperature change was noted for any of the metallic components during MR imaging. However, the metallic components of this device (e.g., halo ring, vertical supports, vest bolts, etc.) vibrated substantially during MR imaging. Furthermore, when the skull pins were held firmly during MR imaging, there was a so-called "drilling" sensation, which could be interpreted as a "burning" effect by the patient. Nevertheless, the skull pins remained cool to the touch throughout the MR procedure (138).

In consideration of the above information, it is inadvisable to permit patients with certain cervical fixation devices to undergo MR procedures using an MTC pulse sequence until this problem can be further characterized to avoid other similar patient responses, regardless of the lack of safety concern related to excessive heating. Other comparable pulse sequences should likewise be avoided when performing MR imaging of patients with halo vests and cervical fixation devices until the precise cause of this problem is determined (102,138). Additionally, all instructions for the use and patient application provided by the halo vest and cervical fixation device manufacturers should be followed, without exception.

Heart Valve Prostheses

Many heart valve prostheses have been evaluated for the presence of attraction to static magnetic fields of MR systems at field strengths of as high as 2.35 T (41,56,62,63,95). Of these, the majority displayed measurable yet relatively minor attraction to the static magnetic field of the MR system used for testing. Because the actual attractive forces exerted on these heart valves were minimal compared to the force exerted by the beating heart (i.e., approximately 7.2 N) (64), an MR procedure is not considered to be hazardous for a patient that has any of the heart valve prostheses already tested. This includes the Starr-Edwards Model Pre-6000 heart valve prosthesis, which was previously suggested to be a potential hazard for a patient undergoing an MR procedure. With respect to clinical MR procedures, there has never been a report of a patient incident or injury related to the presence of a heart valve prosthesis.

Intravascular Coils, Filters, and Stents

Various types of intravascular coils, filters, and stents have been evaluated for safety with MR systems (34,62,65–67,107,110, 111,134), and several demonstrated magnetic field interactions associated with exposure to MR systems. Fortunately, these particular devices typically become incorporated into the vessel wall within 6 weeks after their introduction due to tissue ingrowth. Therefore, it is unlikely they would move or dislodge as a result of being attracted by static magnetic fields of MR systems up to 1.5 T (65). Other similar devices made from nonferromagnetic materials, such as the LGM IVC filter (Vena Tech) used for caval interruption, or the Wallstent biliary endoprosthesis [Schneider (USA), Inc.] used to treat biliary obstruction (111), are safe for patients undergoing MR procedures (107,111,134). It is unnecessary to wait a period after surgery to perform an MR procedure in a patient with a metallic implant that is made from a nonferromagnetic material.

The Guglielmi detachable coil (GDC), used for endovascular embolization, was evaluated for MRI safety (110). Importantly, because of the coiled-shape of the GDC, there exists a potential for excessive heating from induced current to occur during MR imaging. Therefore, a study was performed using *ex vivo* testing techniques to determine the MR compatibility of the Guglielmi detachable coil with respect to magnetic field interactions, heating, and artifacts (110). The results indicate no magnetic field attraction. The temperature increase was mimimal during "worst case" MR imaging and the artifacts involved a mild signal void relative to the size and shape of the GDC. Subsequently, more than 100 patients with GDCs have undergone MR imaging without incident. Other embolization coils made from Nitinol, platinum, or platinum and iridium have been evaluated and found to be safe for patients undergoing MR procedures.

Patients with the specific intravascular coils, filters, and stents listed in the section "List of Items Tested" have had procedures using MR systems with static magnetic fields up to 1.5 T without reported injuries or other problems. Nevertheless, an MR procedure should not be performed if there is any possibility that the intravascular coil, filter, or stent is not positioned properly or firmly in place.

Ocular Implants and Devices

Of the different ocular bioimplants and devices tested, the Fatio eyelid spring, the retinal tack made from martensitic (i.e., ferromagnetic) stainless steel (Western European), the Troutman magnetic ocular implant, and the Unitek round wire eyelid spring were attracted by a 1.5 T static magnetic field (62,96). A patient with a Fatio eyelid spring or round wire eyelid spring may experience discomfort but would probably not be injured as a result of exposure to the magnetic fields of an MR system. Patients have undergone MR procedures with eyelid wires after having a protective plastic covering placed around the globe along with a firmly applied eye patch.

The retinal tack made from martensitic stainless steel and Troutman magnetic ocular implant may injure a patient undergoing an MR procedure although no such case has ever been reported (see section on *Magnetically Activated Implants and Devices* for additional information pertaining to the Troutman magnetic ocular implant).

Orthopedic Implants, Materials, and Devices

Most of the orthopedic implants, materials, and devices evaluated for ferromagnetism are made from nonferromagnetic materials and, therefore, are safe for patients undergoing MR procedures (62). Only the Perfix interference screw used for reconstruction of the anterior cruciate ligament has been found to be highly ferromagnetic (60).

Because this interference screw is firmly imbedded in bone for its specific application, it is held in place with sufficient force to counterbalance it and to prevent movement or dislodgement (60).

Of note is that the presence of the Perfix interference screw causes extensive image distortion during MR imaging of the knee (60). Therefore, one of the other nonferromagnetic interference screws that are available should be used for reconstruction of the anterior cruciate ligament if MR imaging is to be utilized for subsequent evaluation of the knee (60). Patients with each of the orthopedic implants, materials, and devices listed in the section "List of Items Tested" have undergone MR procedures using MR systems with static magnetic fields up to 1.5 T without incident.

Otologic Implants

A patient who has any of the three different cochlear implants listed in the section "List of Items Tested" should not be exposed to the magnetic fields of the MR system because these devices are ferromagnetic (2,3,62,103). Furthermore, these devices are activated by electronic and/or magnetic mechanisms which could be problematic for patients who undergo MR procedures (see section on *Magnetically Activated Implants and Devices* for additional information).

Of the remaining otologic implants that have been evaluated for the presence of ferromagnetism, only the McGee stapedectomy piston prosthesis, made from platinum and chromium-nickel alloy stainless steel, is ferromagnetic (2,3,62). This type of otologic implant has been recalled by the manufacturer, and patients who received these devices have been issued warnings to avoid MR procedures (3). The specific item and lot numbers of the McGee implants that were recalled and considered to be contraindicated for

MR procedures are as follows (personal communication, Winston Geer, Smith & Nephew Richards Inc., Barlett, TN, 1995):

Item No.	Lot No.
14-0330	1W91100, 4UO9690
14-0331	4U09700
14-0332	1W91110, 4U58540, 4U86300
14-0333	4U09710, 1W34390, 2WR4073
14-0334	4U09720, 1W34390, 2WR4073
14-0335	1W34400, 4U09730
14-0336	3U18350, 3U50470, 4UR2889
14-0337	3U18370, 4UR2889
14-0338	3U18390, 4U02900, 4UR1453
14-0339	3U18400, 3U50500
14-0340	3U18410, 3U50500
14-0341	3U41200, 4UR2889

Patent Ductus Arteriosus (PDA), Atrial Septal Defect (ASD), and Ventricular Septal Defect (VSD) Occluders

Metallic cardiac occluders are bioimplants used to treat patients with patient ductus arteriosus (PDA), atrial septal defect (ASD), or ventricular septal defect (VSD) heart conditions. As long as the proper size of the occluder is used, the amount of retention provided by the folded-back, hinged arms of the device is sufficient to keep it in place, acutely. Eventually, tissue growth covers the cardiac occluder and facilitates retention (86).

The metallic PDA, ASD, and VSD occluders tested for ferromagnetism were made from either 304V stainless steel or MP35N. The occluders made from 304V stainless steel were "weakly" ferromagnetism whereas those made from MP35N were nonferromagnetic (86). Patients with cardiac occluders made from 304V stainless steel may undergo MR procedures approximately 6 weeks after placement of these devices, to allow tissue growth to provide additional retentive force, unless there is a concern about the retention of one of these bioimplants. Patients with cardiac occluders made from MP35N (i.e., a nonferromagnetic alloy) may undergo MR procedures any time after placement of these bioimplants (86).

Pellets and Bullets

The majority of pellets and bullets tested for MRI safety are composed of nonferromagnetic materials (69,70). Ammunition that proved to be ferromagnetic tended to be manufactured in foreign countries and/or used for military applications (69,70). Because pellets, bullets, and shrapnel may be contaminated with ferromagnetic materials, the risk vs. benefit of performing an MR procedure in a patient should be carefully considered as well as whether or not the metallic object is located near a vital anatomic structure, with the assumption that the object is likely to be ferromagnetic. Shrapnel typically contains steel and, therefore, presents a potential hazard for patients undergoing MR procedures (69,70). In an effort to reduce lead poisoning in "puddling" type ducks, the federal government requires many of the eastern United States to use steel shotgun pellets instead of lead (70). The presence of steel shotgun pellets presents a potential hazard to patients undergoing MR procedures and causes severe imaging artifacts at the immediate position of these metallic objects (70). In one case, a small metallic BB located in a subcutaneous site caused painful symptoms in a patient exposed to the magnetic fields of the MR system. In consideration of this information, MR users should exercise caution whenever deciding to perform an MR procedure in patients with pellets, bullets, or shrapnel.

Smugar et al. (118) conducted an investigation to determine if neurologic problems developed in patients with intraspinal bullets or bullet fragments during an MRI performed at 1.5 T. Patients were queried during scanning for symptoms of discomfort, pain, or change in neurologic status. Additionally, detailed neurologic examinations were performed prior to MRI, post MRI, and at the patients' discharge. Based on their findings, Smugar et al. concluded patients with complete spinal chord injury may undergo MRI if they have intraspinal bullets or fragments without concern for affecting their physical or neurological status. Thus, metallic fragments in the spinal canals of paralyzed patients represent only a relative contraindication to MRI.

Penile Implants

Several different types of penile implants and prostheses have been evaluated for MRI safety. Of these, two (the Duraphase and Omniphase models) demonstrated substantial ferromagnetic qualities when exposed to a 1.5 T static magnetic field of an MR system (44). Although it is unlikely a penile implant would severely injure a patient undergoing an MR procedure because of the relative strength of the magnetic field interactions, in consideration for the manner in which this type of device is utilized, it would undoubtedly be uncomfortable for the patient. For this reason, subjecting a patient with one of these implants to an MR procedure is inadvisable.

Vascular Access Ports and Catheters

Vascular access ports and catheters are bioimplants commonly used to provide long-term vascular administration of chemotherapeutic agents, antibiotics, analgesics and other medications (104,105). These devices are implanted typically in a subcutaneous pocket over the upper chest wall with the catheters inserted either in the jugular, subclavian, or cephalic vein. Smaller vascular access ports, which are less obtrusive and tend to be tolerated better, have also been designed for implantation in the arms of children or adults, with vascular access via an antecubital vein.

Vascular access ports have a variety of inherent features (e.g., a reservoir, central septum, and catheter) and are constructed from various types of materials including stainless steel, titanium, silicone, and various forms of plastic. Because of the widespread use of vascular access ports and associated catheters and the high probability that patients with these devices may require MR procedures, it was important to determine the MR-compatibility of these bioimplants.

Three of the implantable vascular access ports and catheters evaluated for compatibility with MR procedures showed measurable attraction to the static magnetic fields of the MR systems used for testing, but the forces were considered to be minor relative to

Information Concerning Implants and Materials

the *in vivo* application of these implants (53,104,105). Therefore, MR procedures are safe to perform in a patient that may have one of the vascular access ports or catheters listed in the section "List of Items Tested."

With respect to MR imaging and artifacts, in general, the vascular access ports that produce the least amount of artifact in association with MR imaging are made entirely from nonmetallic materials, whereas the ones that produce the greatest amount of artifact are composed of metal(s) or have metal in an unusual shape (e.g., the OmegaPort Access devices) (104,105). Some manufacturers of vascular access ports have decided to make devices entirely from nonmetallic materials under the assumption this is required for the device to be "MRI-compatible." In fact, several manufacturers produced brochures stating their devices allow "distortion free imaging" or "will not obscure important structures" during MRI.

In one marketing brochure, an MR image is shown that is color-enhanced such that the artifact caused by a "competitors" metallic vascular access port appears to be inordinately large, whereas the manufacturer's plastic vascular access port caused essentially no distortion of the image (unpublished observations, F. Shellock, 1994). This misrepresents the actual MRI compatibility issue and promotes a marketing claim that is without support from a diagnostic MR imaging standpoint.

Even the so-called "MRI compatible" or "MRI ports" made entirely from nonmetallic materials are, in fact, seen on the MR images because they contain silicone (104,105). The septum portion of each of the vascular access ports typically is made from silicone. Using MRI, the Larmor precessional frequency of fat is close to that of silicone (i.e., 100 Hz at 1.5 T). Therefore, silicone used in the construction of vascular access ports may be observed on MR images with varying degrees of signal intensity depending on the pulse sequence selected for imaging (104,105).

Manufacturers of nonmetallic vascular access ports have not addressed this finding during advertising and marketing of their products. On the contrary, vascular access ports made from nonmetallic materials are claimed to be "MRI-compatible" and be "invisible" on MR images. However, if a radiologist did not know this type of vascular access port was present in a patient, the MR signal produced by the silicone component of the device could be considered an abnormality, or at the very least, present a confusing image. For example, this may present a diagnostic problem in a patient being evaluated for a rupture of a silicone breast implant, because silicone from the vascular access port may be misread as an "extracapsular silicone implant rupture."

In more general terms, it is improbable an artifact produced by the presence of any of the tested metallic vascular access ports or catheters will detract from the diagnostic capabilities of MR imaging. The extent of the artifact is relatively minor and, as such, is unlikely to obscure any important anatomical structures by its presence. MR imaging examinations of the chest, where most vascular access ports are typically implanted in a subcutaneous pocket, account for less than 5% of diagnostic studies performed using this imaging modality.

Finally, an important issue related to the construction of vascular access ports should be discussed. These devices are typically made of metal to guard against piercing the injection site by repetitive insertions of needles used to refill the reservoir. Additionally, repeated needle access of a plastic reservoir compared to a metal reservoir may perturb the functional integrity and long-term durability of the vascular access port, as suggested by recent evidence (unpublished findings, 1994). This could result in embolization by fragmented plastic pieces or a reduced ability to properly flush the vascular access port. Therefore, vascular access ports with reservoirs made from metal or other similar hard material may be more acceptable for use in a patient compared to those made from plastic (104,105).

Future developments in vascular access port technology will produce devices that are activated and regulated electronically as well as being programmable. The presence of this type of vascular access port would likely be contraindicated for a patient undergoing an MR procedure.

Miscellaneous

Many different miscellaneous bioimplants, materials, devices, and objects have been tested for ferromagnetic qualities. The cerebral ventricular shunt tube connector (type unknown) and Sophy adjustable pressure valve are devices that have substantial attraction to the static magnetic field of the MR system and, therefore, may present a hazard to a patient undergoing an MR procedure. Another metallic bioimplant, the O-ring washer vascular marker, displayed only slight ferromagnetic qualities and, therefore, does not pose a risk to any patient examined by an MR system.

Kanal and Shabaini (120) tested various types of firearms in the MR environment. Each of these firearms exhibited strong ferromagnetism and two of the six discharged reproducibly. The authors concluded that a firearm in MR environment should be unloaded before removal or any other manipulation of the firearm is attempted (120).

Contraceptive diaphragms were attracted strongly by the 1.5 T static magnetic field used for testing these devices (62). However, MR procedures have been performed in patients with these devices, and they did not complain of any sensation related to movement of the diaphragms. Therefore, the presence of a diaphragm is not believed to be a contraindication for a patient undergoing an MR examination. There is a remote possibility, however, that the contraceptive properties of the diaphragm may be affected if it is inadvertently moved during an MR procedure (62).

After performing a craniotomy, bone flaps are typically fixed with wire, suture material, or small plates and screws. Problems related to cranial bone flap fixation after craniotomy are more common with the trend for performing smaller craniotomies that are frequently utilized for minimally invasive surgical procedures. The use of small plates and screws for fixation of cranial bone flaps has improved the overall attachment process and end result. However, this technique requires a considerable amount of time and expense compared to using wire and suture techniques. Recently, a special metallic implant system, named the Craniofix (Aesculap, Inc., South San Francisco, CA) has been developed for refixation of cranial bone flaps after craniotomy (142). Tests conducted to assess magnetic field interaction, heating, and artifacts indicated the presence of the clamps used for the cranial bone flap fixation system will present no risk to the patient in the MRI environment (142). Furthermore, the quality of the diagnostic MR images is more than acceptable, particularly if conventional spin echo or fast spin echo pulse sequences are used primarily for imaging.

Conventional surgical techniques that rely on direct viewing of the surgical field have several limitations, including the fact that the surgical exposures are typically larger than necessary (i.e., to provide the surgeon adequate room to assess the involved anatomy). Additionally, there may be the need to remove normal tissue to have access to deep targets. Whereas the implementation of endoscopy has resulted in the ability to perform minimally invasive surgery, there are also limitations associated with this technique. The limitations are primarily due to the reduced visibility afforded by the relatively small field of view of the endoscope, such that there is impaired depth perception and an inability of the endoscopist to relate the visual field of the endoscope to the surrounding anatomy. The performance of endoscopy in combination with MR guidance has been proposed to offer several advantages including a dramatic improvement in the visualization and orientation of the endoscope, an ability to appreciate complex three-dimensional anatomy in immediate and remote anatomic areas, and a reduction in procedure-related morbidity (143–150).

The lack of commercially available, MR-compatible medical devices and instruments has obviously hindered the widespread implementation of MR-guided procedures, particularly those involving the use of somewhat complicated instruments like endoscopes. Commercially available endoscopes are constructed from materials that are ferromagnetic. Therefore, the use of these devices is restricted in the MR environment primarily due to the substantial magnetic field attraction and production of large imaging artifacts (unpublished observations, F. G. Shellock, 1997). The presence of metallic medical devices not only creates possible hazards for the patient undergoing the procedure, but also may produce problems for the physician using the instrument in the MR environment. Recently, endoscopes and other support devices (Greatbatch Scientific, Clarence, NY) have been specially designed for use in the MR environment (126, 150). *Ex vivo* testing indicated no apparent concerns of movement or dislodgement, excessive heating, or substantial artifacts that would prevent the safe and successful use of these devices for MR-guided endoscopy (126).

The Deponit patch (Schwarz Pharma, Milwaukee, WI), which is a nitroglycerin transdermal delivery system, contains aluminum. Aluminum is nonferromagnetic and, therefore, not attracted to the static magnetic field of an MR system. However, at least one patient wearing one of these patches received a second-degree burn during an MR imaging procedures (personal communication, Robert E. Mucha, Schwarz Pharma, Milwaukee, WI, 1995). Therefore, it is recommended that a patient using this or similar transdermal delivery system with a metallic component have the patch removed prior to an MR procedure to prevent a potential burn. A new patch should be applied after the examination is completed with the knowledge of the treating or prescribing physician (personal communication, Robert E. Mucha, Schwarz Pharma, Milwaukee, WI; 1995). This information is now included in the product insert for the Deponit patch.

Implanted upper eyelid weights typically made from gold are used to prevent injury in patients with facial nerve paralysis (147). Some of these individuals may require postoperative evaluation for recurrent lateral skull base disease or for other reasons. A study conducted by Marra et al. (147) reported that is is safe to perform MRI in patients with these implants using a 1.5 T MR system.

MR-guided biopsy, therapeutic, and minimally invasive surgical procedures are important clinical applications that are performed on conventional, open-architecture, or the "double donut" MR systems specially designed for this work (148-150). These procedures present challenges with regard to the instruments and devices needed to support these interventions. Obviously, metallic surgical instruments and other devices potentially pose hazards (e.g., "missile effects") or other problems (i.e., image distortion that can obscure the area of interest and either affect adequate visualization of the abnormality or prevent performance of the procedure) that must be addressed to apply MR-guided techniques effectively.

Various manufacturers have used "weakly" ferromagnetic, non-ferromagnetic or nonmetallic materials to make special instruments for interventional MR procedures (131). At least one manufacturer has used ceramic material as a means of constructing prototype devices that include scalpels, cranial drill bits, scissors, and tweezers which have been determined to be MR-compatible (108). Ceramic instruments were shown to have particularly good qualities for the MR environment insofar as there was no magnetic field attraction, negligible heating, and no substantial image distortion determined by the *ex vivo* testing techniques for this material (108).

Other medical products and devices have been developed with metallic components that are either entirely nonferromagnetic (e.g., stereotactic headframe, Compass International, Inc., Rochester, MN) or made from metals that are minimally attracted (e.g., laryngoscopes with lithium batteries, Greatbatch Scientific, Clarence, NY) to the magnetic fields of MR systems. Appendix I provides a comprehensive list of vendors who have developed medical products specifically for interventional MR procedures. These products can be used for MR-guided procedures, as long as these devices have been thoroughly evaluated using accepted MRI safety and compatibility testing techniques and are utilized according to their intended applications.

MR Procedures and Patients with Electrically Activated Implants and Devices

In general, the U.S. Food and Drug Administration (FDA) requires labeling of MR systems to indicate that patients with electrically activated implants or devices should not undergo MR procedures. The electromagnetic fields used by MR systems may interfere with the operation of the devices and there is a possibility the patient could be injured. Examples of electrically activated implants and devices include cardiac pacemakers, implantable cardioverter defibrillators, external hearing aids, cochlear implants, neurostimulators, bone-growth stimulators, and implantable electronic drug infusion pumps. In addition, there are several experimental implants and devices currently undergoing clinical trials that incorporate electrically activated mechanisms. Recently, several implants and devices have been tested for MR safety and, as a result, specific guidelines and recommendations have been developed to permit the safe use of MR procedures in patients with certain electrically activated implants and devices.

Cardiac Pacemakers. Pacemakers are crucial implanted devices for many patients with heart conditions and have served to maintain quality of life and substantially reduce morbidity for these individuals. The first cardiac pacemaker was implanted in 1958. Since then, more than 2 million patients have had cardiac pacemakers implanted. Each year over 100,000 patients in the United States and an additional 100,000 in other parts of the World receive pacemakers for treatment of heart rhythm disturbances.

Cardiac pacemakers are the most common electrically activated implants found in patients that may be referred for MR procedures. Unfortunately, the presence of a cardiac pacemaker is considered a strict contraindication for patients referred for MR procedures (115). The effects of MR systems on the function of a cardiac pacemaker are variable and dependent on several factors including the type of cardiac pacemaker, the static magnetic field strength of the MR system, and the specific type of imaging conditions being used (i.e., the anatomic region imaged, the type of surface coil used, the pulse sequence, etc.) (93,94,97,98,115).

A commonly posed question is whether or not MR procedures may be safely performed under any conditions on patients with implanted cardiac pacemakers. Pacemakers present potential problems to patients undergoing MR procedures from several mechanisms, including (93,94,97,98,115):

1. movement of the pacemaker due to the strong static magnetic field of the MR system;

2. modification of the function of the pacemaker, temporarily and/or permanently, by the static magnetic field of the MR system;

3. heating induced in the pacemaker leads due to the time varying (RF) magnetic fields of the MR system during the imaging process; and

4. voltages and currents induced in the pacemaker leads and/or myocardium during the MR procedure process by the time varying RF and/or the gradient magnetic fields.

Recent work has been performed in this area (personal communication, Rod Gimble, M.D., Cleveland Clinic, 1996). A survey revealed at least two dozen patients with pacemakers have been placed in MR systems, either intentionally or inadvertently. There appears to be documentation that at least six of these patients have died. The cause of death is unknown in these cases.

Much has been written in the radiologic literature about the static field of the MR system closing the reed switches of many pacemakers. These switches close in static fields as low as 15 gauss. Nevertheless, all that reed switch closure accomplishes is placing the pacemaker into an asynchronous mode. A predetermined fixed pacing rate takes over during the time period the reed switch is activated. However, this does not explain why patients would experience cardiac distress or death in MR systems. In fact, thousands of patients are placed into asynchronous mode each day in outpatient visits to cardiologists offices as their pacemakers are interrogated as part of their routine pacemaker maintenance program. Thus, it would appear this often-quoted reed switch activation by the static magnetic field of the MR system may not be the cause of adverse patient outcomes in the MR environment.

There have been several studies in which laboratory dogs as well as human subjects have been tachyarrhythmic and/or hypotensive during MR imaging. It is possible the cause may be the induction of voltages or currents within the pacemaker-lead-myocardial loop that is sufficient to induce action potentials or contraction of the myocardium and an electrical, as well as physiologic, systole. In fact, some cardiologists reported they observed cardiac pacing at the selected repetition time (TR) of the MR imaging procedure. The accuracy of this statement is unclear in light of multislice and/or multiecho and/or spin echo MR imaging protocols, etc. (e.g., radiofrequency cycling rates in spin echo imaging sequences are greater than that determined by the selected TR even in single slice acquisitions). Nevertheless, rapid pacing rates that yield cardiac outputs that are not compatible with sustaining life seem to be responsible as the cause of death in some of the pacemaker patients that underwent MR procedures. Interestingly, with the RF field turned on and the gradients turned off, rapid pacing was still observed.

Electrically Activated Implants and Devices

Heating of the pacemaker/pacing leads during MR imaging is also potentially problematic and thermal injury to the endocardium or myocardium must be considered a possible adverse outcome if RF power is transmitted in the vicinity of the pacemaker and/or its leads. Notably, heating of pacemaker leads and electrodes during MR imaging is a realistic problem. Thermal injury must be considered as a possible adverse outcome if RF power is transmitted in the direct vicinity of the device or its attached components. A recent investigation by Achenbach et al. (132), reported it was possible for electrodes exposed to MR imaging under certain conditions in a 1.5 Tesla MR system to have temperature increases of up to 63.1°C within 90 sec of scanning.

In consideration of all of the above, without an integrated and coordinated approach with cardiology, knowledgeable personnel from radiology, and informed consent from the patient, it should still be considered contraindicated to permit any patient with a cardiac pacemaker to enter the MR environment.

However, it is possible this will change as more knowledge is acquired about this issue and as more information becomes available defining which patients may be safely imaged with MR systems and under what specific conditions. Various theories do suggest it may be possible to perform MR procedures safely in certain patients (such as patients who are not pacemaker dependent) with certain pacemakers. For example, for MR procedures in which the body coil is not used for RF excitation and where continuous physiologic monitoring is being performed throughout the examination, it may be acceptable to perform an examination using MR imaging.

Most of the prior studies on MR-related pacemaker interactions were performed with older MR systems (i.e., virtually a decade ago) using weaker RF transmitter and gradient subsystems. Therefore, there may be reason to hesitate regarding the substantially stronger RF transmitters and gradient magnetic fields more commonly used in many present-day MR systems. This is especially so for the echo planar imaging MR systems with gradient fields that may be five to 10 times more powerful than the ones available 14 years ago. Perhaps at these gradient magnetic field levels the issue of induced arrhythmias secondary to change in gradient magnetic fields needs to be re-examined.

A letter to the editor published in *PACE* indicated a patient who was not pacemaker-dependent was examined by MR imaging after having his cardiac pacemaker "disabled" during the procedure (94). Although this patient did not experience any apparent discomfort and the cardiac pacemaker was not damaged (94), it is inadvisable to perform this type of maneuver routinely on patients with cardiac pacemakers because of the potential to encounter the various aforementioned hazards.

In the event of exposure (inadvertent or intentional) of a patient with an implanted cardiac pacemaker to the static and/or time-varying magnetic fields of an MR imaging system, it would be prudent to have the functionality of the pacemaker checked and verified by a cardiologist. Furthermore, if possible, it would be advisable to have the functionality affirmed by the manufacturer of the particular pacing device.

Retained Cardiac Pacing Wires and Temporary Cardiac Pacing Wires. Certain patients may have cardiac pacing wires that are not connected to a pulse generator. Careful consideration must be given to these cases prior to performance of MR procedures. For example, there may be retained cardiac pacing wires in a patient associated with a prior cardiac surgery. Additionally, a patient may have temporary cardiac pacing wires placed for use with an external cardiac pacemaker (pulse generator) typically utilized to treat cardiac arrhythmias, bradycardia, or tachycardia.

A recent study by Hartnell et al. (151) reported patients with retained temporary epicardial pacing wires, cut short at the skin (i.e., after they were no longer used post-surgically), did not experience any changes in baseline electrocardiographic rhythms or experience any symptoms during MR procedures. This investigation is particularly important because the presence of retained pacing wires was previously considered to be a relative contraindication for MR procedures due to the theoretical risk of inducing current which, in turn, could produce arrhythmias in patients. A study by Hartnell et al. (151) utilized 1.0 and 1.5 T MR systems operating with conventional pulse sequences. Therefore, it would be prudent to use similar MR techniques and parameters as Hartnell et al. (151) in patients with temporary pacing wires until additional investigations are conducted using imaging methods that use faster gradient magnetic fields or more sophisticated imaging techniques.

Recent work was conducted to assess temporary pacing wires with regard to the MR environment. An *ex vivo* assessment of magnetic field interactions, artifacts, and heating associated with the presence of the temporary pacing wires was performed on the following temporary pacing wires (note that this information is specific to these two types of temporary pacing wires, only):

(1) Temporary Cardiac Pacing Wire, TPW-62, 0 (3.5 metric), (316L SS), Ethicon, Inc., Somerville, NJ and
(2) Temporary Cardiac Pacing Wire With Wave, TPW92, 2-0 (3.0 metric), (316L SS), Ethicon, Inc., Somerville, NJ.

Based on two *ex vivo* tests performed to assess magnetic field interactions, there should be no risk with respect to movement or dislodgement for the temporary cardiac pacing wires that were tested for a patient undergoing an MRI procedure using an MR system with a static magnetic field of 1.5 Tesla or less. That is, the portion of the temporary cardiac pacing wire that shows magnetic field interactions (i.e., the straight wire portion) is outside of the patient's body and will be maintained in a fixed position using tape or other similar method during exposure to the MRI environment. The findings from the artifact evaluation indicate the presence of the temporary cardiac pacing wires should not greatly affect the diagnostic use of MR imaging, as long as the area of interest is not in the exact same position where the temporary cardiac pacing wires are located. The experiment demonstrated relatively minor temperature increases in the temporary cardiac pacing wires that are considered to be physiologically inconsequential. Furthermore, the overall test results do not indicate a hazard or risk to a patient with one of the evaluated temporary pacing wires, if the patient undergoes an MR procedure in an MR system of 1.5 Tesla or less. In addition, the exposure to RF energy cannot exceed a whole body averaged specific absorption rate of 1.1 W/kg and conventional pulse sequences must be used.

The specific recommended guidelines for performing an MR procedure in a patient with temporary cardiac pacing wires are, as follows:

(1) The temporary cardiac pacing wires must be disconnected from the pulse generator prior to the MR procedure (i.e., the patient cannot be paced during the MR procedure). The pulse generator should not be placed in the MRI environment.

(2) The ends of the temporary cardiac pacing wires (i.e., the straight leads that connect to the pulse generator) should be taped together to insulate them. The ends of the temporary cardiac pacing wires should be securely attached to the patient using adhesive or other type of tape.

(3) The temporary cardiac pacing wires should be placed on the patient in a "straight line" configuration, without any loops and fixed in this position using tape or other means.

(4) Static Magnetic Field of the MR System and Pulse Sequences: MRI should only be performed using MR systems with static magnetic fields of 1.5 Tesla or less and conventional techniques. Standard spin echo, fast spin echo, and gradient echo pulse sequences may be used. Pulse sequences (e.g., echo planar techniques) or conditions that produce exposure to high levels of RF energy (i.e., exceeding a whole body averaged specific absorption rate of 1.1 W/kg) or exposure to gradient fields that exceed 20 Tesla/second, or any other unconventional MRI technique should be avoided.

(5) Gradient Magnetic Fields of the MR Systems: Pulse sequences (e.g., echo planar imaging techniques or other rapid imaging pulse sequences), gradient coils or other techniques and procedures that exceed a gradient magnetic field of 20 Tesla/sec must not be used for MRI procedures. The use of unconventional or nonstandard MRI techniques must be avoided.

(6) Radiofrequency (RF) Fields of the MR Systems: MRI procedures must not exceed exposures to RF fields greater than a whole body averaged specific absorption rate (SAR) of 1.1 W/kg. The use of unconventional or non-standard MRI techniques must be avoided.

(6) MRI Artifacts: Artifacts for temporary cardiac pacing wires have been characterized using a 1.5 Tesla MR system and various pulse sequences. In general, the artifact size is dependent on the type of pulse sequence used for imaging, the direction of the frequency encoding direction, and the size of the field of view.

(7) Similar to the performance of other MR procedures, the patient should be continuously observed during the MR procedure and instructed to report any unusual sensations to the MR system operator. If these occur, the MR procedure should be discontinued.

Implantable Cardioverter Defibrillators. Implantable cardioverter defibrillators (ICDs) are medical devices designed to automatically detect and treat episodes of ventricular fibrillation, ventricular tachycardias, and bradycardia. When an arrhthmia is detected, the device can deliver defibrillation, cardioversion, antitachycardia pacing, or bradycardia pacing therapy. Each year over 35,000 ICDs are implanted in patients throughout the world. ICDs are most often used to treat patients with sustained arrhythmias that are refractory to antiarrhythmic pharmacologic treatment (115,152).

An ICD uses a programmer that has an external magnet to test the battery charger and to activate and deactivate the system (115,152). Deactivation of an ICD is accomplished by holding a magnet over the device for approximately 30 seconds. It has occurred accidentally as a result of patients encountering magnetic fields in their home and workplace (152). For example, deactivation of ICDs has occurred in patients from exposure to the magnetic fields found in stereo speakers, bingo wands, and 12 volt starters (152).

Magnetic fields of MR systems would have a similar effect on ICDs and, therefore, patients with these devices should avoid exposure to the MR environment. In addition, since ICDs also have electrodes that are placed in the myocardium, patients should not undergo MR procedures because of the previously mentioned risks related to the presence of these conductive materials.

Additional information on performing MR procedures in patients with cardiac pacemakers or implantable cardioverter defibrillators is provided in the section titled, *Safety Considerations for the Extremity MR System.*

Hearing Aids and Cochlear Implants. External hearing aids are included in the category of electrically-activated bioimplants that may be found in patients referred for MR procedures. The magnetic fields used for MR procedures can easily damage these devices. Fortunately, external hearing aids can be readily identified and removed from the patients or individuals to allow them to safely enter the MR environment or to undergo MR procedures.

Some types of cochlear implants employ a relatively strong magnet used in conjunction with an external component to align and retain a radiofrequency transmitter coil on the patient's head (36,116,117,119). The magnet may also be used to provide sufficient transmission quality between the external transmitter and internal receiver (117). Other types of cochlear implants are electronically activated (36,116,117,119). Consequently, MR procedures are typically contraindicated in patients with this classification of implant because of the possibility of injuring the patient and/or damaging or altering the function of the cochlear implant. In general, visitors or other individuals should be prevented from entering the MR environment if they have a cochlear implant. Recently, investigations have been conducted to determine if there are any situations during which a patient with a cochlear implant could undergo MR imaging (116,117,119,153,154).

Two studies have been performed to evaluate the safety of performing MR procedures in patients with specially modified devices: the Nucleaus Mini-22 Cochlear Implant and the Multichannel Auditory Brainstem Implant (153,154). Tests were conducted to assess the operation of the implants in the MR environment as well as magnetic field attraction, artifacts, induced current, and heating during MR imaging (153,154). The reports indicate the results were acceptable with a large margin of safety as long as specific recommendations contained within the product labeling were adhered to (153,154).

In vitro experiments were conducted to determine MR safety for the cochlear implant, the Combi 40/40+ multichannel system (MedEl, Innsbruck, Austria)(116). This cochlear implant underwent testing associated with 0.2 and 1.5 Tesla MR systems. According to the results of the experiments, partial demagnetization of the cochlear implant occurred within the 1.5 Tesla MR system, while the 0.2 Tesla MR system produced no alteration in the magnetic component of this implant (116). Partial demagnetization could be avoided by orienting the patient's head parallel to the magnetic field of the 1.5 Tesla MR system. In general, electromagnetic interference related to the use of the 1.5 Tesla MR system remained within acceptable limits (116). Of the greatest concern were the relative amounts of magnetic field translational attraction and torque acting on the cochlear implant, which have important implications for the safe performance of MR procedures using the 1.5 Tesla MR system. MR safety issues were minimal with the use of the 0.2 Tesla MR system. The authors recommended that MR imaging may be performed in patients with the Combi 40/40+

multichannel system only if there is a strong medical indication (116).

Additional *in vitro* work was conducted on the Combi 40/40+ cochlear implant to determine MRI safety within a wide range of clinical applications using a 1.5 Tesla MR system (117). Torque, translational force, demagnetization, artifacts, induced voltages, and heating were assessed under extreme MR imaging conditions. While most studied parameters were evaluated to assess the electromagnetic interferences with the cochlear implant remained within acceptable limits, the torque on the internal magnet was problematic (117). In addition, external stabilization of this cochlear implant is necessary for a patient undergoing an MR procedure. The overall test findings for the Combi 40/40+ cochlear implant indicated that an MR procedure should only be performed if there is a strong medical necessity (117). An assessment of the relative risks involved versus the risk of not providing the diagnostic capabilities of MR imaging for the specific patient is required.

Implanted Neurostimulators. The incidence of patients receiving implanted neurostimulators for treatment of various forms of neurological disorders is increasing. There are two types of neurostimulators (155):

1. *Passive receivers.* Neurostimulators that receive radiofrequency energy magnetically coupled from an external device by means of a coil placed over the implanted device.

2. *Hermetically encased pulsed generators.* Neurostimulators that contain a battery and are programmed by an external device to produce the various stimulus parameters.

Because of the specific design and intended function of neurostimulators, the electromagnetic fields used for MR procedures may produce problems with the operation of these devices. Malfunction of a neurostimulator that results from exposure to the electromagnetic fields of an MR system may cause discomfort or pain to the patient (155). In extreme cases, damage to the nerve fibers at the

Electrically Activated Implants and Devices

site of the implanted electrodes of the neurostimulator may also occur (155). Therefore, the present policy regarding neurostimulators is patients with these devices should not undergo MR procedures for reasons similar to those indicated for patients with cardiac pacemakers and ICDs.

Six different models of implantable neurostimulators have been evaluated in an *ex vivo* manner in conjunction with 0.35 and 1.5 T MR systems (155). The authors of this study reported that "patients with certain types of implanted neurostimulators can be scanned safely under certain conditions" (155). Unfortunately, this investigation had several limitations. For instance, it did not assess the effects of the variety of pulse sequences used for MR imaging that may substantially alter the function of an implantable neurostimulator. Additionally, an *in vivo* evaluation was not performed (155).

Implantable pulse generators also are currently used for suppression of upper extremity tremors in patients who are diagnosed with essential tremor or parkinsonian tremor not adequately controlled by medications, or where the tremor constitutes a significant functional disability. For example, the Medtronic Activa Tremor Control System is an implantable, multiprogrammable quadripolar system that delivers electrical stimulation to the thalamus to control tremor. It is comprised of the Itrel II Model 7424 Implantable Pulse Generator that has electronic circuitry and a battery, which are hermetically sealed in a titanium case. The operation of this device is supported by a console programmer and a control magnet (Product information, Medtronic Neurological, Minneapolis, MN, 1997).

The product insert information for the Medtronic Activa Tremor Control System indicates patients with this system should not be exposed to the electromagnetic fields produced by MRI. Besides possible dislodgement, heating, and induced voltages in the pulse generator and/or lead, an induced voltage through the pulse generator or lead may cause uncomfortable "jolting" or "shocking" levels of stimulation for the patient in the MR environment. Of note is there have been two anecdotal reports from patients using deep brain stimulation for the treatment of chronic pain who experienced speech problems, temporary sensation of visual light, dizziness and nausea when exposed to MRI (Product information, Medtronic Neurological, Minneapolis, MN, 1997). Due to the associated problems, performing MR procedures in patients with this or a similar device is not recommended. Furthermore, the FDA indicates the presence of this implantable neurostimulator is a contraindication for a patient undergoing an MR procedure. Therefore, MR procedures should not be performed in patents with implantable neurostimulators until the FDA reviews the available safety data and provides the proper approval or recommendations.

The neurostimulators, ITREL II and ITREL III (Medtronic, Minneapolis, MN) underwent safety testing during MR imaging at 0.2, 0.25, and 1.5 Tesla (120). While no apparent heating occurred, the reed switches of these devices were activated. Furthermore, local electrical effects were not determined for these particular implanted neurostimutors, indicating that additional work remains to be conducted to assess other potential problems that may pose a risk to the patient undergoing MR imaging (120).

The neurostimulator, NeuroCybernetic Prosthesis, NCP, Pulse Generator, Model 100 (Cyberonics, Webster, TX) recently received approval for an MR safe labeling claim from the United States Food and Drug Administration, allowing MR procedures to be conducted in patients according to the following strict guidelines (Product label, NeuroCybernetic Prosthesis, NCP, Pulse Generator, Model 100, Cyberonics, Webster, TX):

(1) MRI should not be done with the MR body coil.
(2) Static magnetic fields should be ≤ 2.0 Tesla.
(3) The whole body averaged specific absorption rate must be <1.3 W/kg for a 70 kg patient.
(4) The time varying field should be <10 Tesla/sec.
(5) Magnetic and RF fields produced by MRI may change the pulse generator settings (e.g., change to reset parameters), activate the device, and injure the patient.

Electrically Activated Implants and Devices

Implantable Bone Fusion Stimulators. The implantable spinal fusion stimulator (Electro-Biology, Inc., Parsippany, NJ) is designed for use as an adjunct therapy to a spinal fusion procedure (133). The implantable spinal fusion stimulator consists of a direct current generator with a lithium iodine battery and solid-state electronics encased in a titanium shell, partially-coated with platinum that acts as an anode (133). The generator weighs 10 grams and has the following dimensions: 45 mm × 22 mm × 6 mm. Two nonmagnetic silver/stainless steel leads insulated with silastic provide a connection to two titanium electrodes that serve as the cathodes. A continuous 20 microamp current is produced by this device. The cathodes are comprised of insulated wire leads that terminate as bare wire leads, which are embedded in pieces of bone grafted onto the lateral aspects of fusion sites (133). The generator is implanted beneath the skin and muscle near the vertebral column and provides the full-rated current for approximately 24 to 26 weeks (133).

The use of this implant provides a faster consolidation of the bone grafts, leading to higher fusion rates and improved surgical outcomes, along with a reduced need for orthopedic instrumentation (133). To date, the implantable spinal fusion device has been utilized successfully to increase the probability of bone fusion in more than 70,000 patients (133).

Recent studies using excessively high electromagnetic fields under highly specific experimental conditions and modeling scenarios for the lumbar/torso area (i.e., high-field-strength MR system, excessive exposures to RF fields, excessive exposures to gradient magnetic fields, etc.) demonstrated the implantable spinal fusion stimulator will not present a hazard to a patient undergoing MR imaging with respect to movement, heating, or induced electric fields during the use of conventional MR techniques (121–123,131, 156). Additionally, there was no evidence of malfunction of the implantable spinal fusion stimulator based on *in vitro* and *in vivo* experimental findings (133). Notably, these studies addressed the use of conventional pulse sequences and parameters with an acknowledgement that echo planar techniques or imaging parameters that require excessive RF power will have different implications and consequences for the patient with an implantable spinal fusion stimulator.

To date, MR examinations have been performed in over 120 patients (conceivably, using MR imaging conditions that involved a wide-variety of imaging parameters and conditions) with implantable spinal fusion stimulators, with no reports of substantial adverse events (based on recent review of data obtained through the Freedom of Information Act and unpublished observations, Simon BJ, Electro-Biology, Inc., Parsippany, NJ, 1998). Furthermore, the manufacturer of this implant and the Food and Drug Administration have not received complaints of injuries associated with the presence of this device in patients undergoing MR procedures.

In a recent *in vivo* study (133), there were no reports of immediate or delayed (minimum of one month follow up) adverse events from patients with implantable spinal fusion stimulators who underwent MR imaging at 1.5 T. Each patient was visually inspected following the MRI study and there was no evidence of excessive heating (i.e., change in skin color or other similar response). One patient indicated a sensation of "warming" felt at the site of the stimulator, however, this feeling was described as minor and the MR examination was completed without further indication of unusual sensations or problems (133). Of further note is there were no reports of excessive heating or neuromuscular stimulation in association with the presence of the implantable spinal fusion stimulators in patients that underwent MR imaging (133).

Chou et al. (156) conducted a thorough investigation of the effect of heating of the implantable spinal fusion stimulator associated with MR imaging. This work was performed using a full-sized human phantom during MR procedures involving a relatively high exposure to RF energy (i.e., at whole body averaged specific absorption rates of approximately 1.0 W/kg) (156). Fiber-optic thermometry probes were placed at various positions on and near the cathodes, leads and the stimulator for each experiment to record temperature changes. The phantom used by Chou et al. (156) did not include the effects of blood flow, which would help dissipate heating that may occur during MR imaging and, therefore, further represent an excessive RF exposure condition.

With the implantable spinal fusion stimulator in place and the leads intact, the maximum temperature rise after 25 minutes of scanning occurred at the center of the stimulator and was less than 2.0°C (156). The temperature rise at the cathodes was less than 1.0°C. When the simulator and leads were removed, the maximum temperature rise was less than 1.5°C, recorded at the tip of the electrode with insignificant temperature changes occurring at the cathode (156). These temperature changes are within physiologically acceptable ranges for the tissues where the implantable spinal fusion stimulator is implanted, especially considering that the temperatures for muscle and subcutaneous tissues are at levels that are known to be several degrees below the normal core temperature of 37°C.

Chou et al. (156) also investigated heating of the tips of broken leads of the implantable spinal fusion stimulator (this device was the same as that which underwent testing in the present study). Temperature changes occurred in localized regions that were within a few millimeters of the cut ends of the leads, with maximum temperature increases that ranged from 11 to 14.0°C (156). If these levels of temperatures occurred during MR imaging, the amount of possible tissue damage would be comparable in characteristics and clinical significance to a small electrosurgical lesion and would likely occur in the scar tissue that typically forms around the implanted leads. Additionally, the potential for tissue damage is only theoretical and a brief temperature elevation around a broken lead, over an approximated volume of 2 to 3 mm radius may not be clinically worse than the scar tissue that forms over the leads during implantation. Fortunately, broken leads are rare, occurring in approximately 10 out of the 70,000 devices implanted over the last ten years (personal communication, Simon BJ, Electro-Biology, Inc.).

Based on the available findings from the various investigations that have been conducted, RF energy-induced heating during MR imaging does not appear to present a major problem for a patient with the implantable spinal fusion stimulator, as long as there is no broken lead. The integrity of the leads should be assessed using a radiograph prior to the MR procedure. In general, it is believed the implantable spinal fusion stimulator is safe for patients undergoing MR procedures following specific guidelines. Recommended guidelines for conducting an MR examination in a patient with the implantable spinal fusion stimulator are, as follows:

(1) The cathodes of the implantable spinal fusion stimulator should be positioned a minimum of 1 cm from nerve roots to reduce the possibility of nerve excitation during an MR procedure.

(2) Plain films should be obtained prior to MR imaging to verify that there are no broken leads present for the implantable spinal fusion stimulator. If this cannot be reliably determined, then the potential risks and benefits to the patient requiring MR imaging must be carefully assessed in consideration of the possibility of the potential for excessive heating to develop in the leads of the stimulator.

(3) MR imaging should be performed using MR systems with static magnetic fields of 1.5 T or less and conventional techniques including spin-echo, fast spin-echo, and gradient echo pulse sequences should be used. Pulse sequences (e.g., echo planar techniques) or conditions that produce exposures to high levels of RF energy (i.e., exceeding a whole body averaged specific absorption rate of 1.0 W/kg) or exposure to gradient fields that exceed 20-T/second, or any other unconventional MR technique should be avoided.

(4) Patients should be continuously observed during MR imaging and instructed to report any unusual sensations including any

feelings of warming, burning, or neuromuscular excitation or stimulation.

(5) The implantable spinal fusion stimulator should be placed as far as possible from the spinal canal and bone graft since this will decrease the likelihood that artifacts will affect the area of interest on MR images.

(6) Special consideration should be given to selecting an imaging strategy that minimizes artifacts if the area of interest for MR imaging is in close proximity to the implantable spinal fusion stimulator. The use of fast spin-echo pulse sequences will minimize the amount of artifact associated with the presence of the implantable spinal fusion stimulator.

Electronically Activated, Implantable Drug Infusion Pump. A programmable, implantable drug infusion pump (SynchroMed, Medtronic) used for automatic delivery of antineoplastic agents, morphine, or antispasticity drugs was tested for compatibility with MR systems (157). This device has ferromagnetic components, a magnetic switch, and is programmed by telemetry (157). The presence of these aforementioned features in a device is usually considered reason for the device being designated as contraindicated for patients undergoing MR procedures (115). Nevertheless, the function and integrity of this implantable drug infusion pump was evaluated for compatibility with a 1.5 T MR system (157). The authors concluded that MR imaging was accurate and safe as long as it was understood that the area of interest must be at least 10 cm from the pump and that there was an awareness that a temporary cessation of infusion (i.e., the roller pump rotor appeared to be frozen when the infusion pump was inside the MR system) occurs during the MR procedure (157).

There were several limitations of the assessment performed to determine compatibility of the electronic SynchroMed drug infusion pump (note there is also a vascular access port called Synchromed that is an osmotic, passive device that is acceptable for patients undergoing MR procedures) with MR systems. For example, only a *single* volunteer was examined by MR imaging and the infusion pump was placed *externally* on this subject (157). It is possible that substantially different test results would have been obtained with an implanted infusion pump.

Additionally, only conventional T1-weighted, proton density-weighted, and T2-weighted pulse sequences were evaluated using a single type of MR system. Different MR systems operating with different static magnetic field strengths and operating with different RF fields or using pulse sequences that require higher levels of radiofrequency energy (i.e., fast spin echo) or more severe gradient magnetic fields (i.e., fast gradient echo or echo planar techniques) were not assessed. Therefore, it is probably premature, considering the limited testing procedures conducted to date, to recommend MR imaging may be performed safely on patients with the electronic SynchroMed infusion pump. Furthermore, the manufacturer has not received approval to label this device ''MR-safe.''

Magnetically Activated Implants and Devices

Various types of implants and devices incorporate magnets as a means of activating the implant. The magnet may be used to retain the implant in place (e.g., certain prosthetic devices), to guide a ferromagnetic object into a specific position, to change the operation of the implant, or to program the device (62,115,165–167). Because there is a high likelihood of perturbing the function of magnetically activated implants, demagnetizing the implants, or displacing the implants, MR procedures typically should not be performed in patients with these implants or devices (29,50,115). However, in some cases, patients with magnetically activate implants and devices may undergo MR procedures as long as certain precautions are followed (166,167).

Implants and devices that use magnets (e.g., certain types of dental implants, magnetic sphincters, magnetic stoma plugs, magnetic ocular implants, otologic implants, and other similar prosthetic devices) may be damaged by the magnetic fields of the MR systems which, in turn, may necessitate surgery to replace or reposition them (50,62,75,165). For example, Schneider et al. (165) reported the MRI scan is capable of demagnetizing the permanent magnet associated with an otologic implant (i.e., the Audiant magnet). Obviously, this has important implications for the patient undergoing an MR procedure.

Whenever possible, and if this can be done without risk to the patient (i.e., from the retained magnetic "keeper" or similar component), a magnetically activated implant or device (e.g., an externally applied prosthesis or magnetic stoma plug) should be removed from the patient prior to the MR procedure. This will permit the examination to be performed safely. Knowledge of the specific aspects of the magnetically activated implant or device is essential to recognize potential problems and to guarantee that an MR procedure may be performed on a patient without problems or an injury.

Extrusion of an eye socket magnetic implant in a patient imaged with a 0.5 T MR system has been described (75). This type of magnetic prosthesis is used in a patient after enucleation. A removable eye prosthesis adheres with a magnet of opposite polarity to a permanent implant sutured to the rectus muscles and conjunctiva by magnetic attraction through the conjunctiva (75). This "magnetic linkage" enables the eye prosthesis to move in a coordinated fashion with that of normal eye movement. In the reported incident, the static magnetic field of the MR system produced sufficient attraction of the ferromagnetic portion of the magnetic prosthesis to cause it to extrude through the tissue, thus, injuring the patient (75).

Certain dental prosthetic appliances utilize magnetic forces to retain the implant in place (50). The magnet may be contained within the prosthesis and attached to a ferromagnetic post implanted in the mandible or vise versa (50). An MR procedure may be performed safely in a patient with this type of dental magnet appliance as long as it has been determined that it is properly attached to supporting tissue.

Patients with hydrocephalus or other disorders are often treated with a percutanous adjustable pressure valve which may have a magnetically activated component that allows a change to be made to the resistance required to open the valve (166,167). This is accomplished using an externally applied magnet (166,167). Pressure adjustable valves permit noninvasive readjustment of the opening pressure of an implanted shunt to cerebrospinal fluid hydrodynamics (167). Changing the resistance of this type of valve by MR-induced dysfunction of this implant without recognizing it could cause problems, including acute hydrocephalus, for the patient (166,167). Currently, it is recommended that patients with the percutaneous adjustable pressure valves (e.g., the Sophy or Codman-Medos programmable valves) have the specific valve checked immediately before and after the MR procedure to determine if exposure to the MR system caused a change in the valve setting (166,167). If a change occurred as a result of the MR procedure, the neurosurgeon or other individual responsible for the medical management of the patient and familiar with the operation of this type of device should be notified to reset the percutaneous adjustable pressure valve to its original setting (166,167). Fortunately, there are no known risks or hazards associated with the Sophy or Codman-Medos programmable valves with respect to movement, torque or heating in the MR environment (166,167).

Screening Patients with Metallic Foreign Bodies

All patients or other individuals with a history of being injured by a metallic foreign body such as a bullet, shrapnel, or other type of metallic fragment or object should be thoroughly evaluated prior to admission to the area of the MR system (55,59,88). This is particularly important because serious injury may occur as a result of movement or dislodgement of the metallic foreign body as it is attracted by the magnetic field of the MR system.

The relative risk of injury is dependent on the ferromagnetic properties of the foreign body, the geometry and dimensions of the object, the strength of the static magnetic field, and the strength of the spatial gradient of the MR system. Additionally, the potential for injury is related to the amount of force with which the object is fixed within the tissue (i.e., counter-force or retention force) and whether or not it is positioned in or adjacent to a particularly sensitive site of the body. These sensitive sites include vital neural, vascular, or soft tissue structures (55,59,88,115,137).

Any individual with a suspicion of having an intraocular metallic foreign body (e.g., a metal worker exposed to metallic slivers with a history of an eye injury requiring medical attention) should have plain film radiographs of the orbits to determine the presence of a metallic fragment prior to exposure to the MR environment (55,59,88,115). If an individual with a suspected ferromagnetic intraocular foreign body has no history of a prior injury, no previ-

Screening Patiens with Metallic Foreign Bodies

ous or present symptoms, and a plain film series of the orbits does not demonstrate a foreign body, the risk of injury associated with exposure to the MR system is considered to be minimal (55,59,88,115). Of note is that detection of a high-density focus associated with a metal in the ocular region is not always easy. For example, using CT, it is possible to mistake a calcification for a metallic foreign body in the orbit.

A case report illustrates special precautions are needed for screening of adolescent patients prior to MR procedures (137). This paper described an incident in which a 12-year-old patient accompanied by his parent completed all routine procedures prior to preparation for MR imaging of the lumbar spine. The pre-MR examination screening process included the recommendations and questionnaire developed by the Safety Committee of the Society for Magnetic Resonance Imaging (SMRI) (55). The patient and parent provided negative answers to questions regarding prior injury by metallic objects or the presence of a metallic foreign body.

While entering the MR system room, the adolescent patient appeared to be anxious about the examination (137). He was placed in a feet-first, supine position on the scanner table and prepared for MR imaging. The patient became more anxious and restless, shifting his position several times on the table. As the patient was moved slowly toward the opening of the bore of a 1.5 T MR system, he complained of a pressure sensation in his left eye. The MR technologist immediately removed the patient away from the MR system and out of the room (137).

Once again, the patient was questioned regarding any previous eye injuries, and again he denied any history of injury or problems (137). Despite that patient's response, an intraocular foreign body was suspected to be present. To be prudent, plain-film radiographs of the orbits were obtained, with the patient performing upward and downward fixed glazes. These plain films revealed a metallic foreign body in the left orbit, curvilinear in shape and approximately 5 mm in size (137). Fortunately, the patient did not appear to have sustained an injury to the eye during this incident. The patient and parent were counseled regarding the implications of future MR procedures with respect to the possibility of significant eye injury related to movement or dislodgement of the metallic foreign body.

This case clearly demonstrates that routine guidelines and safety protocols may not always be sufficient for evaluation of potential hazardous situations, particularly in adolescents referred for MR procedures. There are possible additional risks involved whenever parents or guardians fill out MR screening forms because children may not be willing to disclose previous injuries or accidents. In consideration of this incident, and to avoid accidents related to the electromagnetic fields used for MR procedures, it is recommended adolescents be provided additional screening that includes private counseling about the hazards associated with the MR environment (137). Furthermore, the technical staff should be educated about these issues.

In addition to being used to detect metallic objects in the ocular region, plain-film radiography may be used when screening a patient for the presence of a metallic object located in other potentially hazardous sites of the body (88,115). Each MR site should establish a standardized policy for screening patients and individuals with suspected metallic foreign bodies. The policy should include guidelines concerning which individuals or patients require evaluation by radiographic procedures and the specific procedure to be performed (i.e., number and type of views, position of the anatomy, etc.). Furthermore, each case should be carefully considered on an individual basis. These precautions should be taken with respect to any type of MR system regardless of the strength of the static magnetic field, type of magnet, and the presence or absence of magnetic shielding (115).

Screening and Protecting Individuals and Patients From "Missile Effect" Injuries

The "missile effect" refers to the capability of the fringe field component of the static magnetic field to attract ferromagnetic objects (e.g., oxygen tanks, tools, etc.) that may be subsequently drawn into the MR system by considerable force (115). The missile effect can pose a significant risk to the patient inside the MR system and/or anyone who is in the path of the ferromagnetic object that is attracted by the magnetic fringe field. In extreme cases, the magnet may need to be "quenched" for high-field-strength MR systems with superconducting magnets or turned-off to extract sizable ferromagnetic objects from the MR systems. This results in substantial financial loss due to down-time, replacement of cryogens, etc. Therefore, a protocol should be established by every MR site for detection of metallic objects prior to allowing individuals or patients to enter into the area of the MR system to avoid injuries or similar problems related to the missile effect (115).

To guard against these catastrophes, the immediate area around the MR system should be clearly demarcated, labeled with appropriate warning signs, and secured by trained staff who are aware of MR-related safety procedures. Furthermore, patients and other individuals who enter the MR system area should be carefully screened for objects that may be involved in the missile effect.

For a patients preparing to undergo MR procedures, all metallic personal belongings (i.e., analogue watches, jewelry, etc.) and devices must be removed as well as clothing items that have metallic fasteners or other metallic components. One of the more effective means of preventing a ferromagnetic object from inadvertently becoming a missile is to require the patient to where a gown. Additionally, accompanying individuals must be required to remove all objects from their pockets and hair before entering the MR area and carefully screened using the same criteria used for patients. Furthermore, patients and other individuals should be thoroughly educated about the potential hazards and problems associated with the magnetic fringe field before entering the area of the MR system.

Nonambulatory patients must enter the area of the MR system using a nonferromagnetic wheelchair or nonferromagnetic gurney. Wheelchairs and gurneys should also be inspected for the presence of a ferromagnetic oxygen tank or other similar components or accessories before allowing the patient into the MR setting. Fortunately, there are several commercially available, MR-safe devices that may be used to transport and support patients to and from the MR system room (115).

Tattoos, Permanent Cosmetics, and Eye Makeup

Prior to undergoing an MR procedure, the patient should be asked if he or she has ever had any type of permanent coloring technique (i.e., tattooing) applied to any part of the body. This includes cosmetic applications such as eyeliner, lip-liner, lip coloring, as well as decorative designs. This question is necessary because of the associated imaging artifacts and, more importantly, because a small number of patients (fewer than 10) have experienced transient skin irritation, cutaneous swelling, or heating sensations at the site of the permanent colorings in association with MR procedures. More recently, there has been one anecdotal report of a patient undergoing MR imaging who complained of a burning sensation at the site where a large tattoo had been applied on his arm using a black pigment.

Investigating the patients' problems due to the presence of tattoos revealed they occurred when pigments containing iron oxide, or other similar ferromagnetic substances, were used (90,91,115). This includes pigments that are especially black or blue in color. Supposedly, certain ferrous pigments used for the tattooing process can interact with the electromagnetic fields used for MR procedures, producing the reported problems (90,91,115).

A recent case report indicated a 24 year old patient experienced a sudden burning pain at the site of a decorative tattoo while undergoing an MR procedure on the lumbar spine using a 1.5 T MR system (135). Swelling and erythema was resolved within 12 hours, with no evident permanent sequela (135). To complete the MR examination, an excision of the tattooed skin with primary closure of the site was performed (135). Apparently, the tattoo pigment used in this case was ferromagnetic, accounting for the symptoms experienced by the patient. Note the authors of this report wrote, "theoretically, the application of a pressure dressing of the tattoo may prevent any tissue distortion due to ferromagnetic pull." (135). However, this was not attempted for this patient. They also indicated, "in some cases, removal of the tattoo may be the most practical means of allowing MRI."

Kanal and Shellock (136) commented on this report in a letter to the editor, suggesting the events were "rather aggressive." Clearly the trauma, expense, and morbidity associated with excision of the tattoo far exceed those which may be associated with ferromagnetic tattoo interactions (136). The demonstration of grossly detectable ferromagnetic characteristics of a tattoo is not new and has been well-known for over a decade. Certainly, the painful sensation experienced by the patient could not be considered a serious adverse event nor warrant the excision of the tattoo. Particularly in consideration of the existence of other imaging modalities that could be used to assess the lumbar spine (computed tomography, myelography, etc.).

Kanal and Shellock (136) recommended the following procedures to prevent potential problems associated with a similar incident: (1) bandage the area with a pressure dressing and immobilize the tattooed skin with sufficient force to prevent motion of the skin upon exposure to the static magnetic field of the MR system; and (2) in the very rare instance where a patient reports ferromagnetic discomfort or pain, have the patient approach the MR system in a manner to minimize both translational and rotational forces by

Tattoos, Permanent Cosmetics, and Eye Makeup

orienting the patient's tattoo parallel to the magnetic lines of force associated with the MR system.

When one considers the many millions of clinical MR procedures that have been conducted in patients over the past 15 years and that only a few individuals have had a minor, short-term difficulty related to the presence of permanent coloring, it is apparent this problem has an extremely low rate of occurrence and relatively insignificant consequences. Any problem performing an MR procedure in a patient that has a tattoo is unlikely to prevent the examination, since the important diagnostic information provided by this imaging modality is typically critical to the care of the patient.

If a patient with a tattoo requires an MR procedure, the individual should be informed of the relatively minor risk associated with the site of the permanent coloring application. In addition, the patient should be requested to advise the MR operator regarding any unusual sensations felt at the site of the tattoo during the MR examination. Patients with tattoos located on extremities or peripheral sites should be positioned in the MR system to avoid direct contact with the body coil or surface coils (e.g., foam rubber pads may be placed in between the site of the tattoo and the coil) to minimize the potential problem. Similar to other patients undergoing MR procedures, patients with tattoos should be closely monitored using visual and auditory means throughout the entire operation of the MR system to ensure their safety.

With respect to eye makeup, there has been a report of a patient that developed eye irritation when her makeup, which contained ferromagnetic particles, became displaced from her eyelid into her eye during exposure to the MR system (91). Therefore, it is necessary to inform individuals with certain types of eye makeup about the potential problems related to the presence of eye makeup and request that they remove it (if appropriate) before undergoing the MR procedure.

Safety Considerations for the Extremity MR System

Extremity MR System. In 1993, a specially-designed, low-field-strength (0.2 T MR system, Artoscan, Lunar Corp., Madison, WI/Esaote, Genoa, Italy) MR system became available for MR imaging extremities. This MR system uses a small-bore permanent magnet to image feet, ankles, knees, hands, wrists, and elbows. The ergonomic design of the extremity MR system is such that the body part of interest is placed inside the magnet bore, with the patient positioned in a seated or supine position (i.e., depending on the body part that is imaged).

The entire extremity MR system weighs approximately 800 kg, has a built-in radiofrequency shield, multiple body-part-specific extremity coils, and 10 mT/m magnetic gradients. A major advantage of this extremity MR system is that it can be sited in a relatively small space (e.g., approximately 100 square feet) without the need for a special power source, magnetic field shielding, or radiofrequency shielding. Currently, this is the only commercially available extremity MR system approved for use in the United States by the FDA. Note MR imaging using the extremity MR system has been demonstrated to provide a sensitive, accurate, and reliable assessment of various forms of musculoskeletal pathology (158–162).

Because of the unique design features of the extremity MR system (which includes a low-field-strength static magnetic field with a relatively small fringe field) and considering how patients are positioned for MR procedures using this device (i.e., only the body part imaged is placed within the magnet bore while the rest of the body remains outside), it was suggested it may be possible to safely image patients with aneurysm clips, even if they are made from ferromagnetic materials. Furthermore, it may be possible to perform extremity MR imaging in patients with cardiac pacemakers or implantable cardioverter defibrillators (ICDs). Therefore, investigations were conducted to specifically evaluate these safety issues (163,164).

Patients with Ferromagnetic Aneurysm Clips. A study was performed to assess the magnetic field interaction for a variety of different aneurysm clips exposed to the 0.2 T extremity MR system (164). The deflection angle test described by New et al. (39) was used for this assessment. Of additional note is that the FDA issued a draft document (Guidance for Testing MR Interaction with Aneurysm Clips, U.S. Department of Health and Human Services, Food and Drug Administration, Center for Devices and Radiological Health, 1996) that also recommends performing the deflection angle test to determine the magnetic characteristics of aneurysm clips. Twenty-two different types of aneurysm clips were evaluated including those made from nonferromagnetic, weakly ferromagnetic, and ferromagnetic materials (i.e., a Heifetz aneurysm clip made from 17-7PH and a Yasargil, Model FD aneurysm clip). The results indicated that none of the aneurysm clips tested displayed substantial magnetic field interaction in association with the 0.2 T extremity MR system (164).

Because of unique design features of the extremity MR system and in consideration of how patients are positioned for MR procedures using this device (i.e., the head does not enter the magnet bore), it is considered safe to perform MR imaging in patients with the specific aneurysm clips that have been evaluated. These findings effectively permit an important diagnostic imaging modality to be used to evaluate the extemities of patients with suspected musculoskeletal abnormalities using the Artoscan MR system. By comparison, various studies reported patients with Heifetz (17-7PH) and Yasargil, Model FD aneurysm clips (i.e., two of the clips evaluated in the study using the Artoscan) should not undergo MR imaging using MR systems with conventional designs because of the strong attraction shown by these aneurysm clips, which would pose a potential hazard to patients (164).

Patients with Cardiac Pacemakers and Implantable Cardioverter Defibrillators. As previously indicated, patients with cardiac pacemakers and implantable cardioverter defibrillators (ICDs) are generally not permitted to undergo MR procedures. However, due to the design of the Artoscan extremity MR system it may be possible to safely perform MRI in patients with these devices. Since the magnetic fringe field of the extremity MR system is contained in close proximity to the 0.2 T magnet and this system has an integrated Faraday cage, only the patient's extremity is predominantly exposed to the MR-related electromagnetic fields when a procedure is performed. Note it would not be possible for the MR system's gradient or RF electromagnetic field to induce currents in a pacemaker or ICD because the patient's thorax (i.e., where the pacemaker or ICD is typically placed) remains outside of the MR system. Therefore, *ex vivo* experiments were conducted on seven different cardiac pacemakers and seven different implantable cardioverter defibrillators manufactured by Medtronic, Inc. (Minneapolis, MN). The following devices were tested:

Device	Name	Model
Pacemaker	Elite II	7086
Pacemaker	Thera D	7944
Pacemaker	Thera D	7960i
Pacemaker	Thera DR	7962i
Pacemaker	Thera SR	8940
Pacemaker	Kappa	400
Pacemaker	Kappa	700
ICD	PCD	7217D
ICD	Jewel	7219D
ICD	Jewel Plus	7220C
ICD	Micro Jewel	7221Cx
ICD	Micro Jewel II	7223Cx
ICD	Prototype	7250G
ICD	Prototype	7271

Magnetic field attraction was assessed relative to the 0.2 T static magnetic field of the extremity MR system. Additionally, the cardiac pacemakers and implantable cardioverter defibrillators were operated with various lead systems attached while immersed in a tank containing physiologic saline. This apparatus was used to simulate the thorax and was oriented in parallel and perpendicular positions relative to the closest part of the MR system to which a patient undergoing an MR procedure would be positioned. MR studies were performed on a phantom using T1-weighted spin echo and gradient echo sequences. Various functions of the pacemakers and ICDs were evaluated before, during, and after MR imaging.

The results of these tests indicate magnetic field attraction did not present problems for the devices (163). The activation of the pacemakers and cardioverter defibrillators did not substantially affect image quality during MR imaging. Most importantly, the operation of the extremity MR system produced no alterations in the function of the cardiac pacemakers and implantable cardioverter defibrillators (163). Therefore, in consideration of these data and in view of how patients are positioned during MRI using the extremity MR system (i.e., the thorax does not enter the magnet bore), it should be safe to perform MRI in patients with the specific cardiac pacemakers and implantable cardioverter defibrillators evaluated in this study (163).

Other types of dedicated extremity MR systems. In 1998, a new dedicated extremity MR system was developed jointly by Esaote and Siemens Medical Systems. This new device allows MR studies to be conducted on each of the aforementioned body parts as well as the shoulder. Understandably, this particular type of MR system does not have the same inherent design features as the previously-described dedicated extremity system and, as such, this new system should not used to conduct MR procedures in patients with ferromagnetic aneurysm clips or cardiac pacemakers and implantable cardioverter defibrillators. Studies are required to determine if this particular dedicated extremity system may be used to perform MR examinations safely in patients with ferromagnetic implants or other similar typically contraindicated devices.

Future Considerations of Bioimplants, Materials, Devices, and Objects

Several types of investigational bioimplants, materials, devices, and objects are presently undergoing clinical trials. These experimental items incorporate electrically, magnetically, or mechanically activated mechanisms that could pose a hazard to patients referred for MR procedures (168–171). For example, a magnetically controlled heart valve has been described that can be activated so it stays open or closed depending on the requirements of the circulatory system. This prosthetic heart valve uses a small electromagnet that surrounds a ferromagnetic disk within the valve mechanism. Movement of the valve is regulated by the field generated by the electromagnet and the resulting force on the disk (168). The operation of this magnetically-controlled heart valve would be seriously compromised if a patient with this implant were exposed to the electromagnetic fields of an MR system.

An endovascular catheter used for aneurysm embolization has been described that utilizes an external magnetic field for guidance of the device (169). Because this device must be retained in the aneurysm and because inadvertent movement by the magnetic fields of an MR system is possible, the presence of this device would likely be contraindicated for a patient referred for an MR procedure.

Another experimental technique used for embolization of blood vessels has been described whereby ferrous particles are introduced

Future Considerations

into the vascular system and guided by an external magnetic field to the site of the abnormality. If this technique of embolization is used in the clinical setting, patients who have undergone this procedure will need to be identified because of potential risks associated with the displacement of the ferrous particles during exposure to the magnetic fields of MR systems.

The clinical applications of magnetic microspheres used for the targeted and controlled release of medications or diagnostic agents to single or multiple organs is being evaluated presently (170). These magnetic microspheres are typically injected into the arterial system near the targeted organ and then subjected to an externally applied magnetic field gradient ranging from 0.55 to 0.8 T to position them in or near the tissue (170). The magnetic fields associated with MR systems would likely disrupt the placement of the magnetic microspheres. Furthermore, the magnetic microspheres may become dislodged from the intended organ. MR procedures should not be performed in patients with magnetic microspheres until the safety implications have been determined.

The remote magnetic manipulation of a small ferromagnetic "seed" used for delivery of drugs, focal hyperthermia, or other treatments to brain tissues has been described (171). This ferromagnetic seed is maneuvered to a precise location within the brain using static magnetic fields at field strengths less than those used for clinical MR procedures. Iatrogenic displacement of the ferromagnetic seed is likely to occur if a patient with one of these bioimplants is subjected to the magnetic fields associated with an MR system.

As previously mentioned, there are various MR systems that are being used on an on-going investigational basis with static magnetic field strengths of 3.0 and 4.0 T. Furthermore, an 8.0 T MR system is now in operation at Ohio State University. Very few of the biomedical implants or devices have been evaluated for safety in association with these MR systems. Therefore, an extremely cautionary approach is required whenever individuals with ferromagnetic objects are examined using these particular high-field-strength MR systems.

Summary

In general, any patient with an electrically, magnetically, or mechanically activated implant, device, material, or object should be excluded from examination by an MR technique unless it has been demonstrated to be unaffected by the electromagnetic fields of the MR system. Certain electrically, magnetically, or mechanically activated implants or devices may be specially designed to be safe or compatible with the MR environment. However, the federal government agencies responsible for the safe operation of MR systems generally indicates whether the implant or device is acceptable for a patient to undergo an MR procedure. This information is usually indicated in the product insert for the object (not in the marketing materials or other promotional information for the medical device). In lieu of this, MR users may rely on the peer-reviewed literature to guide them with respect to the safety of performing MR procedures when a patient has an implant or device.

References

1. Albert DW, Olson KR, Parel JM, et al. Magnetic resonance imaging and retinal tacks. *Arch Ophthalmol* 1990;108:320–321.
2. Applebaum EL, Valvassori GE. Effects of magnetic resonance imaging fields on stapedectomy prostheses. *Arch Otolaryngol* 1985;11:820–821.
3. Applebaum EL, Valvassori GE. Further studies on the effects of magnetic resonance fields on middle ear implants. *Ann Otol Rhinol Laryngol* 1990;99:801–804.
4. Ballock RT, Hajed PC, Byrne TP, et al. The quality of magnetic resonance imaging, as affected by the composition of the halo orthosis. *J Bone Joint Surg* 1989;71-A:431–434.
5. Barrafato D, Henkelman RM. Magnetic resonance imaging and surgical clips. *Can J Surg* 1984;27:509–512.
6. Becker RL, Norfray JF, Teitelbaum GP, et al. MR imaging in patients with intracranial aneurysm clips. *AJR* 1988;9:885–889.
7. Brown MA, Carden JA, Coleman RE, et al. Magnetic field effects on surgical ligation clips. *Magn Res Imag* 1987;5:443–453.
8. Clayman DA, Murakami ME, Vines FS. Compatibility of cervical spine braces with MR imaging: a study of nine nonferrous devices. *AJNR* 1990;11:385–390.
9. Davis PL, Crooks L, Arakawa M, et al. Potential hazards in NMR imaging: heating effects of changing magnetic fields and RF fields on small metallic implants. *AJR* 1981;137:857–860.
10. de Keizer RJ, Te Strake L. Intraocular lens implants (pseudophakoi) and steelwire sutures: a contraindication for MRI? *Doc Ophthalmol* 1984;61:281–284.
11. Dujovny M, Kossovsky N, Kossowsky R, et al. Aneurysm clip motion during magnetic resonance imaging: in vivo experimental study with metallurgical factor analysis. *Neurosurgery* 1985;17:543–548.
12. Planert J, Modler H, Vosshenrich R. Measurements of magnetism-forces and torque moments affecting medical instruments, implants, and foreign objects during magetic resonance imaging at all degrees of freedom. *Med Phys* 1996;23:851–856.

13. ECRI, Health devices alert. A new MRI complication? May 27, 1988.
14. Gegauff A, Laurell KA, Thavendrarajah A, et al. A potential MRI hazard: forces on dental magnet keepers. *J Oral Rehabil* 1990;17:403–410.
15. Go KG, Kamman RL, Mooyaart EL. Interaction of metallic neurosurgical implants with magnetic resonance imaging at 1.5 Tesla as a cause of image distortion and of hazardous movement of the implant. *Clin Neurosurg* 1989;91:109–115.
16. Gold JP, Pulsinelli W, Winchester P, et al. Safety of metallic surgical clips in patients undergoing high-field-strength magnetic resonance imaging. *Ann Thorac Surg* 1989;48:643–645.
17. Hassler M, Le Bas JF, Wolf JE, et al. Effects of magnetic fields used in MRI on 15 prosthetic heart valves. *J Radiol* 1986;67:661–666.
18. Hathout G, Lufkin RB, Jabour B, et al. MR-guided aspiration cytology in the head and neck at high-field strength. *J Magn Res Imag* 1992;2:93–94.
19. Joondeph BC, Peyman GA, Mafee MF, et al. Magnetic resonance imaging and retinal tacks [Letter]. *Arch Ophthalmol* 1987;105:1479–1480.
20. Kagetsu NJ, Litt AW. Important considerations in measurement of attractive force on metallic implants in MR imagers. *Radiology* 1991;179:505–508.
21. Kanal E, Shellock FG, Talagala L. Safety considerations in MR imaging. *Radiology* 1990;176:593–606.
22. Kanal E, Shellock FG. MR imaging of patients with intracranial aneurysm clips. *Radiology* 1993;187:612–614.
23. Kelly WM, Paglan PF, Pearson JA, et al. Ferromagnetism of intraocular foreign body causes unilateral blindness after MR study. *AJNR* 1986;7:243–245.
24. Kuethe DO, Small KW, Blinder RA. Nonferromagnetic retinal tacks are a tolerable risk in magnetic resonance imaging. *Invest Radiol* 1991;26:1–7.
25. Laakman RW, Kaufman B, Hans JS, et al. MR imaging in patients with metallic implants. *AJR* 1985;8:837–840.
26. Leibman CE, Messersmith RN, Levin DN, et al. MR imaging of inferior vena caval filter: safety and artifacts. *AJR* 1988;150:1174–1176.
27. Lemmens JAM, van Horn R, den Boer, et al. MR imaging of 22 Charnley-Muller total hip prostheses. *Fortschr Geb Rontgenstr* 1986;33:311–315.

28. Leon JA, Gabriele OF. Middle ear prothesis: significance in magnetic resonance imaging. *Magn Res Imag* 1987;5:405–406.
29. Liang MD, Narayanan K, Kanal E. Magnetic ports in tissue expanders: a caution for MRI. *Magn Res Imag* 1989;7:541–542.
30. Lissac MI, Metrop D, Brugigrad, et al. Dental materials and magnetic resonance imaging. *Invest Radiol* 1991;26:40–45.
31. Lufkin R, Jordan S, Lylyck P, et al. MR imaging with topographic EEG electrodes in place. *AJNR* 1988;9:953–954.
32. Lyons CJ, Betz RR, Mesgarzadeh M, et al. The effect of magnetic resonance imaging on metal spine implants. *Spine* 1989;14:670–672.
33. Mark AS, Hricak H. Intrauterine contraceptive devices: MR imaging. *Radiology* 1987;162:311–314.
34. Marshall MW, Teitelbaum GP, Kim HS, et al. Ferromagnetism and magnetic resonance artifacts of platinum embolization microcoils. *Cardiovasc Intervent Radiol* 1991;14:163–166.
35. Matsumoto AH, Teitelbaum GP, Barth KH, et al. Tantalum vascular stents: in vivo evaluation with MR imaging. *Radiology* 1989;170:753–755.
36. Mattucci KF, Setzen M, Hyman R, et al. The effect of nuclear magnetic resonance imaging on metallic middle ear prostheses. *Otolaryngol Head Neck Surg* 1986;94:441–443.
37. Mechlin M, Thickman D, Kressel HY, et al. Magnetic resonance imaging of postoperative patients with metallic implants. *AJR* 1984;143:1281–1284.
38. Mesgarzadeh M, Revesz G, Bonakdarpour A, et al. The effect on medical metal implants by magnetic fields of magnetic resonance imaging. *Skeletal Radiol* 1985;14:205–206.
39. New PFJ, Rosen BR, Brady TJ, et al. Potential hazards and artifacts of ferromagnetic and nonferromagnetic surgical and dental materials and devices in nuclear magnetic resonance imaging. *Radiology* 1983;147:139–148.
40. Power W, Collum LMT. Magnetic resonance imaging and magnetic eye implants [Letter]. *Lancet* 1988;2:227.
41. Randall PA, Kohman LJ, Scalzetti EM, et al. Magnetic resonance imaging of prosthestic cardiac valves in vitro and in vivo. *Am J Cardiol* 1988;62:973–976.
42. Roberts CW, Haik BG, Cahill P. Magnetic resonance imaging of metal loop intraocular lenses. *Arch Ophthalmol* 1990;108:320–321.

43. Seiff SR, Vestel KP, Truwit CL. Eyelid palpebral springs in patients undergoing magnetic resonance imaging: an area of possible concern [Letter]. *Arch Ophthalmol* 1991;109:319.
44. Shellock FG, Crues JV, Sacks SA. High-field magnetic resonance imaging of penile protheses: in vitro evaluation of deflection forces and imaging artifacts [Abstract] In: *Society of Magnetic Resonance in Medicine.* Berkeley, CA;1987:915.
45. Shellock FG, Crues JV. High-field-strength MR imaging and metallic bioimplants: an in vitro evaluation of deflection forces and temperature changes induced in large prostheses [Abstract]. *Radiology* 1987;165:150.
46. Shellock FG, Crues JV. High-field strength MR imaging and metallic biomedical implants: an ex vivo evaluation of deflection forces. *AJR* 1988;151:389–392.
47. Shellock FG. MR imaging of metallic implants and materials: a compilation of the literature. *AJR* 1988;151:811–814.
48. Shellock FG, Crues JV. MRI: safety considerations in magnetic resonance imaging. *MRI Decisions* 1988;2:25–30.
49. Shellock FG. Biological effects and safety aspects of magnetic resonance imaging. *Magn Res Q* 1989;5:243–261.
50. Shellock FG. Ex vivo assessment of deflection forces and artifacts associated with high-field strength MRI of "mini-magnet" dental prostheses. *Magn Res Imag* 1989;7(suppl 1):38.
51. Shellock FG, Slimp G. Halo vest for cervical spine fixation during MR imaging. *AJR* 1990;154:631–632.
52. Shellock FG, Schatz CJ, Shelton C, et al. Ex vivo evaluation of 9 different ocular and middle ear implants exposed to a 1.5 Tesla MR scanner. *Radiology* 1990;177:271.
53. Shellock FG, Meeks T. Ex vivo evaluation of ferromagnetism and artifacts for implantable vascular access ports exposed to a 1.5 T MR scanner [Abstract]. *J Magn Res Imag* 1991;1:243.
54. Shellock FG, Schatz CJ. High-field strength MR imaging and metallic otologic implants. *AJNR* 1991;12:279–281.
55. Shellock FG, Kanal E, SMRI Safety Committee. Policies, guidelines, and recommendations for MR imaging safety and patient management. *J Magn Res Imag* 1991;1:97–101.
56. Shellock FG, Swengros-Curtis J. MR imaging and biomedical implants, materials, and devices: an updated review. *Radiology* 1991;180:541–550.

57. Shellock FG. Safety considerations in MR imaging of biomedical implants and devices. In: Thrall J, ed. *Current practice in radiology.* Philadephia: Decker/Mosby-Year Book, 1992.
58. Shellock FG, Litwer C, Kanal E. MRI bioeffects, safety, and patient management: A review. *Rev Magn Res Imag* 1992;4:21–63.
59. Shellock FG, Crues JV. Safety aspects of MRI in patients with metallic implants or foreign bodies: absolute and relative contraindications. *Appl Radiol* 1992;Nov:44–47.
60. Shellock FG, Mink JH, Curtin S, et al. MRI and orthopedic implants used for anterior cruciate ligament reconstruction: assessment of ferromagnetism and artifacts. *J Magn Res Imag* 1992;2:225–228.
61. Shellock FG, Myers SM, Schatz CJ. Ex vivo evaluation of ferromagnetism determined for metallic scleral "buckles" exposed to a 1.5 T MR scanner. *Radiology* 1992;185:288–289.
62. Shellock FG, Morisoli S, Kanal E. MR procedures and biomedical implants, materials, and devices: 1993 update. *Radiology* 1993;189:587–599.
63. Soulen RL, Budinger TF, Higgins CB. Magnetic resonance imaging of prosthetic heart valves *Radiology* 1985;154:705–707.
64. Soulen RL. Magnetic resonance imaging of prosthetic heart valves [Letter]. *Radiology* 1986;158:279.
65. Teitelbaum GP, Bradley WG, Klein BD. MR imaging artifacts, ferromagnetism, and magnetic torque of intravascular filters, stents, and coils. *Radiology* 1988;166:657–664.
66. Teitelbaum GP, Ortega HV, Vinitski S, et al. Low artifact intravascular devices: MR imaging evaluation. *Radiology* 1988;168:713–719.
67. Teitelbaum GP, Raney M, Carvlin MJ, et al. Evaluation of ferromagnetism and magnetic resonance imaging artifacts of the Strecker tantalum vascular stent. *Cardiovasc Intervent Radiol* 1989;12:125–127.
68. Teitelbaum GP, Lin MCW, Watanabe AT, et al. Ferromagnetism and MR imaging: safety of cartoid vascular clamps. *AJNR* 1990;11:267–272.
69. Teitelbaum GP, Yee CA, Van Horn DD, et al. Metallic ballistic fragments: MR imaging safety and artifacts. *Radiology* 1990;175:855–859.
70. Teitelbaum GP. Metallic ballistic fragments: MR imaging safety and artifacts [Letter]. *Radiology* 1990;177:883.

71. To SYC, Lufkin RB, Chiu L. MR-compatible winged infusion set. *Comput Med Imaging Graph* 1989;13:469–472.
72. Watanabe AT, Teitelbaum GP, Gomes AS, et al. MR imaging of the bird's nest filter. *Radiology* 1990;177:578–579.
73. White DW. Interation between magnetic fields and metallic ossicular prostheses. *Am J Otol* 1987;8:290–292.
74. Williamson MR, McCowan TC, Walker CW, et al. Effect of a 1.5 Tesla magnetic field on Greenfield filters in vitro and in dogs. *Angiology* 1988;12:1022–1024.
75. Yuh WTC, Hanigan MT, Nerad JA, et al. Extrusion of a eye socket magnetic implant after MR imaging examination: potential hazard to a patient with eye prosthesis. *J Magn Res Imag* 1991;1:711–713.
76. Zheutlin JD, Thompson JT, Shofner RS. The safety of magnetic resonance imaging with intraorbital metallic objects after retinal reattachment or trauma [Letter]. *Am J Ophthalmol* 1987;103:831.
77. FDA stresses the need for caution during MR scanning of patients with aneurysm clips. In: Medical Devices Bulletin, Center for Devices and Radiological Health. March, 1993;11:1–2.
78. Klucznik RP, Carrier DA, Pyka R, Haid RW. Placement of a ferromagnetic intracerebral aneurysm clip in a magnetic field with a fatal outcome. *Radiology* 1993;187:855–856.
79. Lufkin R, Layfield L. Coaxial needle system of MR- and CT-guided aspiration cytology. *J Comput Assist Tomogr* 1989;13:1105–1107.
80. Lufkin R, Teresi L, Hanafee W. New needle for MR-guided aspiration cytology of the head and neck. *AJR* 1987;149:380–382.
81. Bellon EM, Haacke EM, Coleman PE, et al. MR artifacts: a review. *Magn Res Imag* 1984;2:41–52.
82. Pusey E, Lufkin RB, Brown RKJ, et al. Magnetic resonance imaging artifacts: mechanism and clinical significance. *Radio Graphics* 1986;6:891–911.
83. Kanal E, Shellock FG. The value of published data regarding MR compatibility of metallic implants and devices. *AJNR* 1994;15:1394–1396.
84. Food and Drug Administration. Magnetic resonance diagnostic device: panel recommendation and report on petitions for MR reclassification. *Federal Registrar* 1988;53:7575–7579.
85. Johnson GC. Need for caution during MR imaging of patients with aneurysm clips [Letter]. *Radiology* 1993;188:287.

References

86. Shellock FG, Morisoli SM. Ex vivo evaluation of ferromagnetism and artifacts for cardiac occluders exposed to a 1.5 Tesla MR system. *J Magn Res Imag* 1994;4:213–215.
87. Dupuy DE, Hartnell GC, Lipsky M. MR imaging of a patient with a ferromagnetic foreign body. *AJR* 1993;160:893.
88. Mani RL. In search of an effective screening system for intraocular metallic foreign bodies prior to MR, an important issue of patient safety. *AJNR* 1988;9:1032.
89. Williams S, Char DH, Dillon WP, et al. Ferrous intraocular foreign bodies and magnetic resonance imaging. *Am J Ophthalmol* 1988;105:398–401.
90. Jackson JG, Acker JD. Permanent eyeliner and MR imaging. *AJR* 1987;49:1080.
91. Lund G, Nelson JD, Wirtschafter JD, Williams PA. Tattooing of eyelids: magnetic resonance imaging artifacts. *Ophthalmic Surgery* 1986;17:550–553.
92. Sacco D, Steiger DA, Bellon EM, et al. Artifacts caused by cosmetics in MR imaging of the head. *AJR* 1987;148:1001–1004.
93. Erlebacher JA, Cahill PT, Pannizzo F, et al. Effect of magnetic resonance imaging on DDD pacemakers. *Am J Cardiol* 1986;57:437–440.
94. Alagona P, Toole JC, Maniscalco BS, et al. Nuclear magnetic resonance imaging in a patient with a DDD pacemaker [Letter]. *PACE* 1989;12:619.
95. Shellock FG, Morisoli SM. Ex vivo evaluation of ferromagnetism, heating, and artifacts for heart valve prostheses exposed to a 1.5 Tesla MR system. *J Magn Res Imag* 1994;4:756–758.
96. Bakshandeh H, Shellock FG, Schatz CJ, Morisoli SM. Metallic clips used for scleral buckling: Ex vivo evaluation of ferromagnetism determined at 1.5 T. *J Magn Res Imag* 1993;3:559.
97. Hayes DL, Holmes DR, Gray JE. Effect of a 1.5 Tesla magnetic resonance imaging scanner on implanted permanent pacemakers. *J Am Coll Cardiol* 1987;10:782–786.
98. Holmes DR, Hayes DL, Gray JE, et al. The effects of magnetic resonance imaging on implantable pulse generators. *PACE* 1986;9:360–370.
99. Moscatel M, Shellock FG, Morisoli S. Biopsy needles and devices: assessment of ferromagnetism and artifacts during exposure to a 1.5 Tesla MR system. *J Magn Res Imag* 1995;5:369–372.

100. Shellock FG, Shellock VJ. Additional information pertaining to the MR-compatibility of biopsy needles and devices. *J Magn Res Imag* 1996;6:411.
101. Fagan LL, Shellock FG, Brenner RJ, Rothman B. Ex vivo evaluation of ferromagnetism, heating, and artifacts of breast tissue expanders exposed to a 1.5 T MR system. *J Magn Res Imag* 1995;5:614–616.
102. Shellock FG. MR imaging and cervical fixation devices: assessment of ferromagnetism, heating, and artifacts. *Magn Res Imag* 1996;14: 1093–1098
103. Nogueira M, Shellock FG. Otologic bioimplants: Ex vivo assessment of ferromagnetism and artifacts at 1.5 Tesla. *AJR* 1995;163:1472–1473.
104. Shellock FG, Nogueira M, Morisoli M. MRI and vascular access ports: ex vivo evaluation of ferromagnetism, heating, and artifacts at 1.5 T. *J Magn Res Imag* 1995;4:481–484.
105. Shellock FG, Shellock VJ. Vascular access ports and catheters tested for ferromagnetism, heating, and artifacts associated with MR imaging. *Magn Res Imag* 1996;14:443–447.
106. Kanal E, Shellock FG, Lewin JS. Aneurysm clip testing for ferromagnetic properties: clip variability issues. *Radiology* 1996;200: 576–578.
107. Kiproff PM, Deeb ZL, Contractor FM, Khoury MB. Magnetic resonance characteristics of the LGM vena cava filter: technical note. *Cardiovasc Intervent Radiol* 1991;14:254–255.
108. Shellock FG, Shellock VJ. Ceramic surgical instruments: evaluation of MR-compatibility at 1.5 Tesla. *J Magn Res Imag* 1996;6:954–956.
109. Shellock FG, Shellock VJ. Evaluation of MR compatibility of 38 bioimplants and devices. *Radiology* 1995;197:174.
110. Shellock FG, Detrick MS, Brant-Zawadski M. MR-compatibility of Guglielmi detachable coils. *Radiology* 1997;203:568–570.
111. Girard MJ, Hahn PF, Saini S, et al. Wallstent metallic biliary endoprosthesis: MR imaging characteristics. *Radiology* 1992;184:874–876.
112. Shellock FG, Kanal E. Burns associated with the use of monitoring equipment during MR procedures. *J Magn Res Imag* 1996;6:271–272.
113. Lewin JS, et al. Needle localization in MR-guided biopsy and aspiration: Effect of field strength, sequence design, and magnetic field orientation. *AJR* 1996;166:1337–1341.
114. Faber SC, Stehline MK, Reiser M. Artifacts of MR-compatible biopsy needles: optimization of pulse sequences dependence on MR-parameters, comparison of different products. Proceedings of the

International Society of Magnetic Resonance in Medicine, Book of Abstracts.1996;3:1741.
115. Shellock FG, Kanal E. *Magnetic resonance: bioeffects, safety and patient management,* 2nd edition. Lippincott-Raven, New York, 1996
116. Teissl C, Kremser C, Hochmair ES, Hochmair-Desoyer IJ. Cochlear implants: in vitro investigation of electromagnetic interference at MR imaging-compatibility and safety aspects. *Radiology* 1998;208:700–708.
117. Teissl C, Kremser C, Hochmair ES, Hochmair-Desoyer IJ. Magnetic resonance imaging and cochlear implants: compatibility and safety aspects. *J Magn Res Imag* 1999;9:26–38.
118. Smugar SS, Schweitzer ME, Hume E. MRI in patients with intraspinal bullets. *J Magn Res Imag* 1999;9:151–153.
119. Ouayoun M, Dupuch K, Aitbenamou C, Chouard CH. Nuclear magnetic resonance and cochlear implant. *Ann Otolaryngol Chir Cervicofac* 1997;114:65–70.
120. Tronnier VM, Stauber A, Hahnel S, Sarem-Aslani A. Magnetic resonance imaging with implanted neurostimulators: an in vitro and in vivo study. *Neurosurgery* 1999;44:118–25.
121. Liem LA, van Dongen VC. Magnetic resonance imaging and spinal cord stimulation systems. *Pain* 1997;70:95–97.
122. Reilly P, Diamant AM. Theoretical evaluation of peripheral nerve stimulation during MRI with an implanted spinal fusion stimulator. *Magn Res Imag* 1997;15:1145–1156.
123. Buechler DN, Durney CH, Christensen DA. Calculation of electric fields induced near metal implants by magnetic resonance imaging switched-gradient magnetic fields. *Magn Res Imag* 1997;15:1157–1166.
124. Shellock FG, Shellock VJ. MR-compatibility evaluation of the Spetzler titanium aneurysm clip. *Radiology* 1998;206:838–841.
125. Shellock FG, Kanal E. Yasargil aneurysm clips: evaluation of interactions with a 1.5 Tesla MR system. *Radiology* 1998;207:587–591.
126. Shellock FG. MR-compatibility of an endoscope designed for use in interventional MRI procedures. *AJR* 1998;71:1297–1300.
127. Shellock FG, Kanal E. Aneurysm clips: Evaluation of MR imaging artifacts at 1.5 Tesla. *Radiology* 1998;209:563–566.
128. Shellock FG, Shellock VJ. Cardiovascular catheters and accessories: Ex vivo testing of ferromagnetism, heating, and artifacts associated with MRI. *J Magn Reson Imag* 1998;8:1338–1342.
129. Kanal E, Shellock FG. Aneurysm clips: effects of long-term and multiple exposures to a 1.5 Tesla MR system. *Radiology* 1999;210:563–565.

130. Shellock FG, Shellock VJ. Metallic marking clips used after stereotactic breast biopsy: ex vivo testing of ferromagnetism, heating, and artifacts associated with MRI. *AJR* (in press).
131. Shellock FG. MRI safety of instruments designed for interventional MRI: assessment of ferromagnetism, heating, and artifacts. *Workshop on New Insights into Safety and Compatibility Issues Affecting In Vivo MR, Syllabus,* 1998; pp. 39.
132. Achenbach S, Moshage W, Diem B, et al. Effects of magnetic resonance imaging on cardiac pacemakers and electrodes. *Am Heart J* 1997;134:467–473.
133. Shellock FG, Hatfield M, Simon BJ, et al. Implantable spinal fusion stimulator: assessment of MRI safety. *AJR* (in press).
134. Shellock FG, Shellock VJ. Stents: Evaluation of MRI safety. *AJR* (in press).
135. Kreidstein ML, Giguere D, Friedberg A. MRI interaction with tattoo pigments: case report, pathophysiology, and management. *Plastic and Reconstructive Surgery* 1997;99:1717–1720.
136. Kanal E, Shellock FG. MRI interaction with tattoo pigments. *Plastic and Reconstructive Surgery* 1998;101:1150–1151.
137. Elmquist C, Shellock FG, Stoller D. Screening adolescents for metallic foreign bodies prior to MR procedures. *J Magn Res Imag* 1996;5:784–785.
138. Hartwell CG, Shellock FG. MRI of cervical fixation devices: Sensation of heating caused by vibration of metallic components. *J Magn Res Imag* 1997;7:771.
139. Malko JA, Hoffman JC, Jarrett PJ. Eddy-current-induced artifacts caused by an "MR-compatible" halo device. *Radiology* 1989;173:563–564.
140. Hua J, Fox RA. Magnetic resonance imaging of patients wearing a surgical traction halo. *J Magn Res Imag* 1996;1:264–267.
141. Kanal E, Shabaini A. Firearm safety in the MR imaging environment. *Radiology* 1994;193:875–876.
142. Shellock FG, Shellock VJ. Evaluation of flap fixation clamps for compatibility with MR imaging. *Radiology* 1998;208:822–825.
143. Scholz M, Deli M, Wildforster U, et al. MRI-guided endoscopy in the brain: a feasibility study. *Minim Invasive Neurosurg* 1996;39:33–37.
144. Seibel RM. Image-guided minimally invasive therapy. *Surg Endosc* 1997;11:154–162.

References

145. Fried MP, Hsu L, Topulos GP, Jolesz FA. Image-guided surgery in a new magnetic resonance suite: preclinical considerations. *Laryngoscope* 1996;106:411–417.
146. Fried MP, Kleefield J, Gopal H, et al. Image-guided endoscopic surgery: results of accuracy and performance in a multicenter clinical study using an electromagnetic tracking system. *Laryngoscope* 1997;107:594–601.
147. Marra S, Leonetti JP, Konior RJ, Raslan W. Effect of magnetc resonance imaging on implantable eyelid weights. *Ann Otol Rhinol Laryngol* 1995;104:448–452.
148. Silverman SG, Collick BD, Figueira MR, et al. Interactive MR-guided biopsy in an open-configuration MR imaging system. *Radiology* 1995;197:175–181.
149. Jolesz FA, Blumenfeld SM. Interventional use of magnetic resonance imaging. *Magn Reson Q* 1994;10:85–96.
150. Jolesz FA, Shtern F. The operating room of the future. *Invest Radiol* 1992;27:326–328.
151. Hartnell GG, et al. Safety of MR imaging in patients who have retained metallic materials after cardiac surgery. *AJR* 1997;168:1157–1159.
152. Bonnet CA, Elson JJ, Fogoros RN. Accidental deactivation of the automatic implantable cardioverter defibrillator. *Am Heart J* 1990;3:696–697.
153. Heller JW, Brackmann DE, Tucci DL, et al. Evaluation of MRI compatibility of the modified nucleus multi-channel auditory brainstem and cochlear implants. *Am J Otol* 1996;17:724–729.
154. Chou H-K, McDougall JA, Can KW. Absence of radiofrequency heating from auditory implants during magnetic resonance imaging. *Bioelectromagnetics* 1995;16:307–316.
155. Gleason CA, Kaula NF, Hricak H, et al. The effect of magnetic resonance imagers on implanted neurostimulators. *PACE* 1992;15:81–94.
156. Chou C-K, McDougall JA, Chan KW. RF heating of implanted spinal fusion stimulator during magnetic resonance imaging. *IEEE Trans Biomed Engineering* 1997;44:357–373.
157. Von Roemeling R, Lanning RM, Eames FA. MR imaging of patients with implanted drug infusion pumps. *J Magn Res Imag* 1991;1:77–81.
158. Barile A, Masiocchi C, Mastantuono M, et al. The use of a "dedicated" MRI system in the evaluation of knee joint diseases. *Clin MRI* 1995;5:79–82.

159. Peterfy CG, Roberts T, Genant HK. Dedicated extremity MR imaging: an emerging technology. *Radiol Clin North Am* 1997;35:1–20.
160. Franklin PD, Lemon RA, Barden HS. Accuracy of imaging the menisci on an in-office, dedicated, magnetic resonance imaging extremity system. *Amer J Sports Med* 1998;25:382–388
161. Masciocchi C, Barile A, Navarra F, et al. Clinical experience of osteoarticular MRI using a dedicated system. *MAGMA* 1994;2:545–550.
162. Shellock FG, Stone K, Crues JV. Development and clinical applications of kinematic MRI of the patellofemoral joint using an extremity MR system. *Med Sci Sport Exerc* (in press)
163. Shellock FG, O'Neil M, Ivans V, et al. Cardiac pacemakers and implantable cardiac defibrillators are unaffected by operation of an extremity MR system. *AJR* 1999;72:165–17.
164. Shellock FG, Crues JV. Aneurysm clips: Assessment of magnetic field interaction associated with a 0.2-T extremity MR system. *Radiology* 1998;208:407–409.
165. Schneider ML, Walker GB, Dormer KJ. Effects of magnetic resonance imaging on implantable permanent magnets. *Am J Otol* 1995;16:687–689.
166. Ortler M, Kostron H, Felber S. Transcutaneous pressure-adjustable valves and magnetic resonance imaging: an ex vivo examination of the Codman-Medos programmable valve and the Sophy adjustable pressure valve. *Neurosurgery* 1997;40:1050–1057.
167. Fransen P, Dooms G, Thauvoy C. Safety of the adustable pressure ventricular valve in magnetic resonance imaging: problems and solutions. *Neuroradiology* 1992;34:508–509.
168. Young DB, Pawlak AM. An electromagnetically controllable heart valve suitable for chronic implantation. *ASAIO Trans* 1990;36:M421–M425.
169. Gaston A, Marsault C, Lacaze A, et al. External magnetic guidance of endovascular catheters with a superconducting magnet: preliminary trials. *J Neuroradiol* 1988;15:137–147.
170. Ranney DF, Huffaker HH. Magnetic microspheres for the targeted controlled release of drugs and diagnostic agents. *Ann NY Acad Sci* 1987;507:104–119.
171. Grady MS, Howard MA, Molloy JA, et al. Nonlinear magnetic stereotaxis: three dimensional in vivo remote magnetic manipulation of a small object in canine brain. *Med Phys* 1990;17:405–415.

List of Items Tested

General Information

As previously-discussed, various articles and lists of implants, materials, devices, and objects tested for interactions with the magnetic fields of MR systems have been published and updated (1-69). The data presented in any list of this type represent a "snapshot in time" for the period indicated and for the specific implants, materials, devices and objects that have been evaluated using the particular technique described in the publication. Therefore, a revised version of the List of Items Tested is necessary. Changes and updated information may occur for a variety of reasons. Manufacturers may change the composition of the implant, material, device, or object without being required to notify or seek new approval from the United States Food and Drug Administration (FDA), as long as the function of the device remains essentially the same. Therefore, MR sites may elect to follow certain guidelines, including contacting the company that manufactured the device to determine if any alterations in component materials occurred since it was tested. This is especially important for those devices that would present a serious hazard to the patient if it was possible that it could be moved or dislodged (e.g., aneurysm clips, otologic implants, etc.) in association with an MR procedure.

Notably, there are now many MR systems with static magnetic field strengths that exceed 2.0 T and most devices or materials were tested at 1.5 T. Very few of the implants, materials, devices, or objects have been assessed to determine the relative amount of attraction to these higher static magnetic fields. It is conceivable a device that exhibited only "mild" or "weak" ferromagnetism in association with a static magnetic field strength of 1.5 T or lower, is now attracted with sufficient force to pose a hazard to a patient or MR user utilizing an MR system that has a static magnetic field strength of 2.0 T or higher. Therefore, careful consideration must be given to each individual implant, material, device or object relative to the particular MR system being used (1-69).

Additional Information For the List of Items Tested and Explanation of Table Footnotes

To properly utilize the information for the implants, materials, devices and objects in the List of Items Tested, particular attention must be given to the highest static magnetic field strength used for testing and the symbols that provide supplemental data and explanations, as follows:

"Highest Field Strength" refers to the highest static magnetic field used for the evaluation of deflection force, magnetic field attraction, or attraction of the various implants, materials, devices, or objects tested.

* Denotes the implant, material, device, or object is considered safe for patents undergoing MR procedures despite being attracted by static magnetic fields. In general, this is due to the fact the attraction was characterized as "mild" relative to the *in vivo* forces present for a given implant, material, device or object. For example, certain prosthetic heart valves were attracted to the magnetic fields of the MR systems, but the attractive forces were considered to be less than the forces exerted on the prosthetic heart valves by the beating heart. Additionally, there may be substantial "retentive" or counterforces present provided by tissue in growth, scarring, or granulation that serve to prevent an implant, material, device, or object from presenting a risk or hazard to the patient. For a device that is used for an MR-guided procedures (e.g., laryngoscope, endoscope, etc.), there may be minimal torque or linear attraction to magnetic fields of MR systems. However, the device is considered to be safe if used in its "intended" manner, as indicated by the manufacturer.

† Ferromagnetic intravascular coils, filters, stents, and cardiac occluders typically become firmly incorporated into the tissue several weeks following placement. Therefore, it is unlikely they will be moved or dislodged by attraction to magnetic fields.

*† Patients with coils, filters, and stents indicated in the attraction/deflection column should wait a minimum 6 weeks prior to an MR procedure to assure firm implantation into the vessel wall if the device is made from ferromagnetic material.

†† Although certain cardiovascular catheters and accessories typically do not exhibit attraction to the magnetic fields of MR systems, there are other mechanisms whereby these devices may pose a hazard to the patient in the MR setting. For example, a triple-lumen thermodilution Swan+Ganz catheter has no attraction to a static magnetic field, however, there was a report of a catheter "melting" in a patient during an MR procedure. Therefore, this catheter and other similar devices would be considered a contraindication for patients undergoing MR procedures.

††† The Deponit, nitroglycerin transdermal delivery system, although not attracted to the static magnetic field of an MR system, has been found to heat excessively during MR imaging. This excessive heating may burn a patient wearing this patch. Therefore,

it is recommended the patch be removed prior to the MR procedure and a new patch applied immediately after the examination.

†††† These devices are attracted to the static magnetic field of the MR system. However, because of the relative amount of attractive force and their *in vivo* use, they are unlikely to pose a hazard in association with dislodgement. The potential risk of performing MR procedures in patients with these devices is related to induced current and excessive heating. Therefore, it is inadvisable to perform MR procedures in patients with these devices.

[a] These halo vests are known to have ferromagnetic components. However, the relative amount of attraction to the magnetic field was not determined.

∞ These devices are considered to be safe for patients undergoing MRI procedures as long as specific guidelines and recommendations are followed. Refer to the pertinent information in the preceding text of this book for the particular device.

N/A, Not applicable. These implants, materials, devices, or objects were tested for ferromagnetism using standardized techniques. However, the data have not been published.

Manufacturer information was provided, if known.

SS, stainless steel.

LIST OF IMPLANTS, MATERIALS, DEVICES, AND OBJECTS TESTED FOR ATTRACTION/DEFLECTION FORCES DURING EXPOSURE TO STATIC MAGNETIC FIELDS

Implant, material, device, or object	Attraction/ deflection	Highest field strength (T)	Reference
Aneurysm and hemostatic clips			
Downs multi-positional (17-7PH)	Yes	1.39	1
Drake (DR 14, DR 21) Edward Weck Triangle Park, NJ	Yes	1.39	1, 2
Drake (DR 16) Edward Weck Triangle Park, NJ	Yes	0.147	1
Drake (301 SS) Edward Weck Triangle Park, NJ	Yes	1.5	2, 3
Gastrointestinal anastomosis clip Auto Suture SGIA (SS) United States Surgical Corp. Norwalk, CT	No	1.5	3
Heifetz (17-7PH) Edward Weck Triangle Park, NJ	Yes	1.89	4, 5
Heifetz (Elgiloy) Edward Weck Triangle Park, NJ	No	1.89	2, 4, 5
Hemoclip, #10 (316L SS) Edward Weck Triangle Park, NJ	No	1.5	3
Hemoclip (tantalum) Edward Weck Triangle Park, NJ	No	1.5	3
Housepian	Yes	0.147	1
Kapp (405 SS) V. Mueller	Yes	1.89	2, 5
Kapp, curved (404 SS) V. Mueller	Yes	1.39	1
Kapp, straight (404 SS) V. Mueller	Yes	1.39	1

Aneurysm and hemostatic clips (continued)

Implant, material, device, or object	Attraction/ deflection	Highest field strength (T)	Reference
Ligaclip, #6 (316L SS) Ethicon, Inc. Sommerville, NJ	No	1.5	3
Ligaclip (tantalum) Ethicon, Inc. Sommerville, NJ	No	1.5	3
Mayfield (301 SS) Codman Randolf, MA	Yes	1.5	3
Mayfield (304 SS) Codman Randolf, MA	Yes	1.89	5
McFadden (301 SS) Codman Randolf, MA	Yes	1.5	2, 3
McFadden Vari-Angle micro clip, straight, 9 mm blade (MP35N) Codman Johnson & Johnson Professional, Inc. Raynham, MA	No	1.5	N/A
McFadden Vari-Angle micro clip, straight fenestrated, 9 mm blade (MP35N) Codman Johnson & Johnson Professional, Inc. Raynham, MA	No	1.5	N/A
Olivercrona	No	1.39	1
Pivot (17-7PH)	Yes	1.89	5
Perneczky Aneurysm Clip 3 mm, straight Zeppelin Chirurgische Instuments Germany	No	1.5	N/A

List of Items Tested

Implant, material, device, or object	Attraction/ deflection	Highest field strength (T)	Reference
Perneczky Aneurysm Clip 9 mm, curved Zeppelin Chirurgische Instruments Germany	No	1.5	N/A
Perneczky Aneurysm Clip 9 mm, straight Zeppelin Chirurgische Instruments Germany	No	1.5	N/A
Perneczky Aneurysm Clip 20 mm, curved Zeppelin Chirurgische Instruments Germany	No	1.5	N/A
Scoville (EN58J) Downs Surgical, Inc. Decatur, GA	No	1.89	2, 5
Spetzler Titanium Aneurysm Clip, straight, 9 mm blade, double turn (C.P. titanium) Elekta Instruments, Inc. Atlanta, GA	No	1.5	59
Spetzler Titanium Aneurysm Clip, straight, 9 mm blade, single turn (C.P. titanium) Elekta Instruments, Inc. Atlanta, GA	No	1.5	59
Spetzler Titanium Aneurysm Clip, straight, 13 mm blade, double turn (C.P. titanium) Elekta Instruments, Inc. Atlanta, GA	No	1.5	59
Spetzler Titanium Aneurysm Clip, straight, 13 mm blade, single turn (C.P. titanium) Elekta Instruments, Inc. Atlanta, GA	No	1.5	59
Stevens (silver alloy)	No	0.15	6
Sugita (Elgiloy) Downs Surgical, Inc. Decatur, GA	No	1.89	2, 5

List of Items Tested

Implant, material, device, or object	Attraction/ deflection	Highest field strength (T)	Reference
Aneurysm and hemostatic clips (continued)			
Sugita AVM Micro Clip (Elgiloy) Mizuho America, Inc. Beverly, MA	No	1.5	N/A
Sugita, straight, large aneurysm clip for permanent occlusion (Elgiloy) Mizuho America, Inc. Beverly, MA	No	1.5	N/A
Sugita, bent, mini aneurysm clip for temporary occlusion (Elgiloy) Mizuho America, Inc. Beverly, MA	No	1.5	N/A
Sugita, bent, standard aneurysm clip for temporary occlusion (Elgiloy) Mizuho America, Inc. Beverly, MA	No	1.5	N/A
Sugita, bent, fenestrated large aneurysm clip for permanent occlusion (Elgiloy) Mizuho Amernica, Inc. Beverly, MA	No	1.5	N/A
Sugita, sideward CVD bayonet, standard aneurysm clip for permanent occlusion Mizuho America, Inc. Beverly, MA	No	1.5	N/A
Sundt AVM, Micro Clip (MP35N) Codman Johnson & Johnson Professional, Inc. Raynham, MA	No	1.5	N/A
Sundt-Kees Multi-Angle (17-7PH) Downs Surgical, Inc. Decatur, GA	Yes	1.89	2, 5
Sundt-Kees Slim-Line, fenestrated, 9 mm blade (MP35N)	No	1.5	N/A

List of Items Tested

Implant, material, device, or object	Attraction/ deflection	Highest field strength (T)	Reference
Codman Johnson & Johnson Professional, Inc. Raynham, MA			
Sundt-Kees, Slim-Line, 9 mm blade, (MP35N)	No	1.5	N/A
Codman Johnson & Johnson Professional, Inc. Raynham, MA			
Sundt Slim-Line, Graft Clip (MP35N)	No	1.5	N/A
Codman Johnson & Johnson Professional, Inc. Raynham, MA.			
Sundt Slim-Line, Temporary Clip, straight, 10 mm blade (MP35N)	No	1.5	N/A
Codman Johnson & Johnson Professional, Inc. Raynham, MA			
Surgiclip, Auto Suture M-9.5 (SS)	No	1.5	3
United States Surgical Corp. Norwalk, CT			
Vari-Angle (17-7PH)	Yes	1.89	5
Codman Randolf, MA			
Vari-Angle McFadden (MP35N)	No	1.89	2, 5
Codman Randolf, MA			
Vari-Angle Micro (17-7PH)	Yes	0.15	2, 6
Codman Randolf, MA			

Aneurysm and hemostatic clips (continued)

Implant, material, device, or object	Attraction/ deflection	Highest field strength (T)	Reference
Vari-Angle Spring (17-7PH) Codman Randolf, MA	Yes	0.15	2, 6
Yasargil, Model FD Aesculap, Inc. South San Francisco, CA	Yes	1.5	N/A
Yasargil, Model FE Aesculap, Inc. South San Francisco, CA	No	1.5	N/A
Yasargil (316 SS) Aesculap, Inc. South San Francisco, CA	No	1.89	5
Yasargil, Model FE 720T, mini, permanent, 7 mm blade, (titanium alloy) Aesculap, Inc. South San Francisco, CA	No	1.5	N/A
Yasargil, Model FE 740T, standard, permanent, 7 mm blade, (titanium alloy) Aesculap, Inc. South San Francisco, CA	No	1.5	N/A
Yasargil, Model FE 748, standard, 9 mm blade, bayonet (Phynox) Aesculap, Inc. South San Francisco, CA	No	1.5	N/A
Yasargil, Model FE 750, 9 mm blade, straight (Phynox) Aesculap, Inc. South Francisco, CA	No	1.5	N/A
Yasargil, Model FE 750T, standard, permanent, 9 mm blade, (titanium alloy) Aesculap, Inc. South San Francisco, CA	No	1.5	N/A

Biopsy needles, markers, and devices

Implant, material, device, or object	Attraction/ deflection	Highest field strength (T)	Reference
Adjustable, Automated Biopsy Gun 6, 13, and 19 mm (304 SS) MD Tech Watertown, MA	Yes	1.5	7
Adjustable, Automated Aspiration Biopsy Gun 10, 15, and 20 mm (304 SS) MD Tech Watertown, MA	Yes	1.5	7
ASAP 16, Automatic 16 G Core Biopsy System 19 cm length (304 SS)	Yes	1.5	7
Automatic Cutting Needle with Dept Markings 14 G, 10 cm length (304 SS) Manan Northbrook, IL	Yes	1.5	7
Automatic Cutting Needle with Ultrasound Tip & Depth Markings 18 G, 16 cm length (304 SS) Manan Northbrook, IL	Yes	1.5	7
Automatic Cutting Needle with Ultrasound Tip & Depth Markings 18 G, 20 cm length (304 SS) Manan Northbrook, IL	Yes	1.5	7
Basic II Hookwire Breast Localization Needle (304 SS) MD Tech Watertown, MA	Yes	1.5	7
Beaded Breast Localization Wire Set 20 G, 2 inch needle with 5-7/8 inch wire (304 SS)	Yes	1.5	7

Biopsy needles, markers, and devices (continued)

Implant, material, device, or object	Attraction/ deflection	Highest field strength (T)	Reference
Inrad Grand Rapids, MI Beaded Breast Localization Wire Set 19 G, 3-1/2 inch needle with 7-7/8 inch wire (304 SS) Inrad Grand Rapids, MI	Yes	1.5	7
Biopsy Gun 13 mm Meadox Oakland, NJ	Yes	1.5	7
Biopsy Gun 25 mm Meadox Oakland, NJ	Yes	1.5	7
Biopsy, Needle 17 G, 10 cm length Meadox Oakland, NJ	Yes	1.5	7
Biopsy Needle 20 G, 15 cm length Meadox Oakland, NJ	Yes	1.5	7
Biopsy Needle 22 G, 15 cm length Meadox Oakland, NJ	Yes	1.5	7
Biopsy Needle 22 G, 15 cm length Cook, Inc. Bloomington, IN	Yes	1.5	7
Biopty-Cut Biopsy Needle 14 G, 10 cm length (304 SS) C.R. Bard, Inc. Covington, GA	Yes	1.5	7

List of Items Tested

Implant, material, device, or object	Attraction/ deflection	Highest field strength (T)	Reference
Biopty-Cut Biopsy Needle 16 G, 16 cm length (304 SS) C.R. Bard, Inc. Covington, GA	Yes	1.5	7
Biopty-Cut Biopsy Needle 18 G, 18 cm length (304 SS) C.R. Bard, Inc. Covington, GA	Yes	1.5	7
Biopty-Cut Biopsy Needle with centimeter markings 18 G, 20 cm length (304 SS) C.R. Bard, Inc. Covington, GA	Yes	1.5	7
Breast Localization Needle 20 G, 5 cm length (304 SS) Manan Northbrook, IL	Yes	1.5	7
Breast Localization Needle 20 G, 7 cm length (304 SS) Manan Northbrook, IL	Yes	1.5	7
Chiba Needle and HiLiter Ultrasound Enhancement 22 G, 3-7/8 inch needle (304 SS) Inrad Grand Rapids, MI	Yes	1.5	7
Coaxial Needle Set Chiba-type Needle 22 G, 5-7/8 inch needle (304 SS) Inrad Grand Rapids, MI	Yes	1.5	7
Coaxial Needle Set Introducer Needle 19G, 2-15/16 inch needle (304 SS) Inrad Grand Rapids, MI	Yes	1.5	7

Implant, material, device, or object	Attraction/ deflection	Highest field strength (T)	Reference

Biopsy needles, markers, and devices (continued)

Implant, material, device, or object	Attraction/ deflection	Highest field strength (T)	Reference
Cutting Needle 14 G, 9 cm length West Coast Medical Laguna Beach, CA	Yes	1.5	7
Cutting Needle 16 G, 17 mm length (304 SS) BIP USA, Inc. Niagara Falls, NY	Yes	1.5	7
Cutting Needle 16 G, 19 mm length (304 SS) BIP USA, Inc. Niagara Falls, NY	Yes	1.5	7
Cutting Needle 18 G, 100 mm length Meadox Oakland, NJ	Yes	1.5	7
Cutting Needle 18 G, 150 mm length Meadox Oakland, NJ	Yes	1.5	7
Cutting Needle 18 G, 9 cm length West Coast Medical Laguna Beach, CA	Yes	1.5	7
Cutting Needle 18 G, 15 cm length West Coast Medical Laguna Beach, CA	Yes	1.5	7
Cutting Needle 19 G, 6 cm length West Coast Medical Laguna Beach, CA	Yes	1.5	7
Cutting Needle 19 G, 9 cm length West Coast Medical Laguna Beach, CA	Yes	1.5	7

List of Items Tested

Implant, material, device, or object	Attraction/ deflection	Highest field strength (T)	Reference
Cutting Needle 19 G, 15 cm length West Coast Medical Laguna Beach, CA	Yes	1.5	7
Cutting Needle 20 G, 9 cm length West Coast Medical Laguna Beach, CA	Yes	1.5	7
Cutting Needle 20 G, 15 cm length West Coast Medical Laguna Beach, CA	Yes	1.5	7
Cutting Needle 20 G, 20 cm length West Coast Medical Laguna Beach, CA	Yes	1.5	7
Cutting Needle & Gun 18 G, 155 mm length Moadox Oakland, NJ	Yes	1.5	7
Hawkins Blunt Needle (304 SS) MD Tech Watertown, MA	Yes	1.5	7
Hawkins III Breast Localization Needle MD Tech Watertown, MA	Yes	1.5	7
Lufkin Aspiration Cytology Needle 20 G, 5 cm length (high nickel alloy) E-Z-Em, Inc. Westbury, NY	No	1.5	9
Lufkin Biopsy Needle 18 G, 5 cm length (high nickel alloy) E-Z-Em, Inc. Westbury, NY	No	1.5	8

Biopsy needles, markers, and devices (continued)

Implant, material, device, or object	Attraction/ deflection	Highest field strength (T)	Reference
Lufkin Biopsy Needle 18 G, 15 cm length (high nickel alloy) E-Z-Em, Inc. Westbury, NY	No	1.5	8
Lufkin Biopsy Needle 22 G, 5 cm length (high nickel alloy) E-Z-Em, Inc. Westbury, NY	No	1.5	8
Lufkin Biopsy Needle 22 G, 10 cm length (high nickel alloy) E-Z-Em, Inc. Westbury, NY	No	1.5	8
Lufkin Biopsy Needle 22 G, 15 cm length (high nickel alloy) E-Z-Em, Inc. Westbury, NY	No	1.5	8
Micromark Clip (316L SS) Biopsys Medical Irvine, CA	No	1.5	62
MReye Chiba Biopsy Needle William Cook Europe A/S Bjaeverskov, Denmark	No	1.5	N/A
MReye Franseen Lung Biopsy Needle William Cook Europe A/S Bjaeverskov, Denmark	No	1.5	N/A
MReye Interventional Needle William Cook Europe A/S Bjaeverskov, Denmark	No	1.5	N/A
MReye Kopans Breast Lesion Localization Needles 21, 20, 19 gauges; 5.0, 9.0, 15.0 lengths William Cook Europe A/S Bjaeverskov, Denmark	No	1.5	N/A

List of Items Tested

Implant, material, device, or object	Attraction/ deflection	Highest field strength (T)	Reference
MRI BioGun 18 G, 10 cm length (high nickel alloy) E-Z-Em, Inc. Westbury, NY	No	1.5	8
MRI Histology Needle 18 G, 5 cm length (high nickel alloy) E-Z-Em, Inc. Westbury, NY	No	1.5	8
MRI Histology Needle 18 G, 15 cm length (high nickel alloy) E-Z-Em, Inc. Westbury, NY	No	1.5	7
MRI Histology Needle 20 G, 5 cm length (high nickel alloy) E-Z-Em, Inc. Westbury, NY	No	1.5	7
MRI Histology Needle 20 G, 7.5 cm length (high nickel alloy) E-Z-Em, Inc. Westbury, NY	No	1.5	8
MRI Histology Needle 20 G, 10 cm length (high nickel alloy) E-Z-Em, Inc. Westbury, NY	No	1.5	8
MRI Histology Needle 20 G, 15 cm length (high nickel alloy) E-Z-Em, Inc. Westbury, NY	No	1.5	8
MRI Lesion Marking System 20 G, 7.5 cm length (high nickel alloy) E-Z-Em, Inc. Westbury, NY	No	1.5	8

List of Items Tested

Implant, material, device, or object	Attraction/ deflection	Highest field strength (T)	Reference
Biopsy needles, markers, and devices (continued)			
MRI Needle (surgical grade SS) Cook, Inc. Bloomington, IN	No	1.5	7
mrt Biopsy Needle Sizes include: 75 mm/14 G 100 mm/14 G 150 mm/14 G 200 mm/18 G 75 mm/18 G 100 mm/18 G 150 mm/18 G 200 mm/18 G (titanium alloy) Daum Medical Baltimore, MD and Schwerin, Germany	No	1.5	N/A
Percucut Biopsy Needle and Stylet 19.5 gauge × 10 cm (316L SS) E-Z-Em, Inc. Westbury, NY	Yes	1.5	7
Percucut Biopsy Needle and Stylet 21 gauge × 10 cm (316L SS) E-Z-Em, Inc. Westbury, NY	Yes	1.5	7
Sadowsky Breast Marking System 20 G, 5 cm length needle and 7 inch hook wire (316 L SS) Ranfac Corporation Avon, MA	Yes	1.5	7
Soft Tissue Biopsy Needle Gun & Needle, (304 SS) Anchor Procducts Co. Addison, IL	Yes	1.5	7

Implant, material, device, or object	Attraction/ deflection	Highest field strength (T)	Reference
Trocar Needle (304 SS) BIP USA, Inc. Niagara Falls, NY	Yes	1.5	7
Trocar Needle, Disposable (SS) Cook, Inc. Bloomington, IN	Yes	1.5	7
Ultra-Core, biopsy needle 16 G, 16 cm length (304 SS) Gainesville, FL	Yes	1.5	7

Breast tissue expanders and implants

Implant, material, device, or object	Attraction/ deflection	Highest field strength (T)	Reference
Becker Expander/Mammary Prosthesis (316L SS) Mentor H/S Santa Barbara, CA	No	1.5	10
Infall, breast implant (inflatable with magnetic port) 3101198 Model Heyerschultzz	Yes	1.5	N/A
Radovan Tissue Expander (316L SS) Mentor H/S Santa Barbara, CA	No	1.5	10
Siltex Spectrum Post-Operatively Adjustable Saline-Filled Mammary Prosthesis (316L SS) Mentor H/S Santa Barbara, CA	No	1.5	10
Tissue expander with magnetic port McGhan Medical Corporation Santa Barbara, CA	Yes	1.5	N/A

Cardiovascular catheters and accessories

Implant, material, device, or object	Attraction/ deflection	Highest field strength (T)	Reference
Opticath Catheter, Model U400 Abbott Laboratories Morgan Hill, CA	No[††]	1.5	61

List of Items Tested

Implant, material, device, or object	Attraction/ deflection	Highest field strength (T)	Reference

Cardiovascular catheters and accessories (continued)

Implant, material, device, or object	Attraction/ deflection	Highest field strength (T)	Reference
Opticath PA Catheter with extra port Abbott Laboratories Morgan Hill, CA	No[††]	1.5	61
Opticath PA Catheter with RV Pacing Port Abbott Laboratories Morgan Hill, CA	No[††††]	1.5	61
Opti-Q SvO_2/CCO Catheter Abbott Laboratories Morgan Hill, CA	No[††]	1.5	61
Oximetric 3, SO_2 Optical Module Abbott Laboratories Morgan Hill, CA	Yes[††]	1.5	61
RV Pacing Lead Abbott Laboratories Morgan Hill, CA	Yes[††]	1.5	61
Swan+Ganz Thermodilution Catheter American Edwards Laboratories Irvine, CA	No[††]	1.5	61
Swan+Ganz Triple-lumen Thermodilution Catheter American Edwards Laboratories Irvine, CA	No[††]	1.5	61
TD Thermodilution Catheter, Flow-directed Thermodilution Pulmonary Artery Catheter Abbott Laboratories Morgan Hill, CA	No[††]	1.5	61
TDQ CCO Catheter, Flow-directed Thermodilution	No[††]	1.5	61

List of Items Tested

Implant, material, device, or object	Attraction/ deflection	Highest field strength (T)	Reference
Continuous Cardiac Output Pulmonary Artery Catheter Abbott Laboratories Morgan Hill, CA	No[††]	1.5	61
Torque-Line Flow-directed Thermodilution Pulmonary Artery Catheter Abbott Laboratories Morgan Hill, CA			
Transpac IV Abbott Laboratories Morgan Hill, CA	No	1.5	61

Carotid artery vascular clamps

Crutchfield (SS) Codman Randolf, MA	Yes*	1.5	11
Kindt (SS) V. Mueller	Yes*	1.5	11
Poppen-Blaylock (SS) Codman Randolf, MA	Yes	1.5	11
Salibi (SS) Codman Randolf, MA	Yes*	1.5	11
Selverstone (SS) Codman Randolf, MA	Yes*	1.5	11

Dental devices and materials

Brace band (SS) American Dental Missoula, MT	Yes*	1.5	3
Brace wire (chrome alloy) Ormco Corp. San Marcos, CA	Yes*	1.5	3

Dental devices and materials (continued)

Implant, material, device, or object	Attraction/ deflection	Highest field strength (T)	Reference
Castable alloy Golden Dental Products, Inc. Golden, CO	Yes*	1.5	12
Cement-in keeper Solid State Innovations, Inc. Mt. Airy, NC	Yes	1.5	12
Dental amalgam	No	1.39	1
Gutta Percha Points	No	1.5	N/A
GDP Direct Keeper, Pre-formed post Golden Dental Products, Inc. Golden, CO	Yes*	1.5	12
Indian Head Real Silver Points Union Broach Co., Inc. New York, NY	No	1.5	N/A
Keeper, pre-formed post Parkell Products, Inc. Farmingdale, NY	Yes*	1.5	1
Magna-Dent, large indirect keeper Dental Ventures of America, Yorba Linda, CA	Yes*	1.5	1
Palladium clad magnet Parkell Products, Inc. Farmingdale, NY	Yes	1.5	13
Palladium/palladium keeper Parkell Products, Inc. Farmingdale, NY	Yes*	1.5	13
Palladium/platinum casting alloy Parkell Products, Inc. Farmingdale, NY	Yes*	1.5	13
Permanent crown (amalgam) Ormco Corp.	No	1.5	3
Stainless steel clad magnet Parkell Products, Inc. Farmingdale, NY	Yes	1.5	13
Stainless steel keeper Parkell Products, Inc. Farmingdale, NY	Yes*	1.5	13

List of Items Tested

Implant, material, device, or object	Attraction/ deflection	Highest field strength (T)	Reference
Silver point Union Broach Co., Inc. New York, NY	No	1.5	3
Titanium clad magnet Parkell Products, Inc. Farmingdale, NY	Yes	1.5	13

ECG Electrodes

Implant, material, device, or object	Attraction/ deflection	Highest field strength (T)	Reference
Accutac ConMed Corp. Utica, NY	No	1.5	N/A
Accutac Diaphoretic ConMed Corp. Utica, NY	No	1.5	N/A
Adult Cloth ConMed Corp. Utica, NY	No	1.5	N/A
Adult ECG Electrode 3-Pack ConMed Corp. Utica, NY	No	1.5	N/A
Adult Foam ConMed Corp. Utica, NY	No	1.5	N/A
Cleartrace 2 ConMed Corp. Utica, NY	No	1.5	N/A
Dyna/Trace ConMed Corp. Utica, NY	No	1.5	N/A
Dyna/Trace Diagnostic ECG Electrode ConMed Corp. Utica, NY	No	1.5	N/A
Dyna/Trace Mini ConMed Corp. Utica, NY	No	1.5	N/A
Dyna/Trace Stress ConMed Corp. Utica, NY	No	1.5	N/A

List of Items Tested

Implant, material, device, or object	Attraction/ deflection	Highest field strength (T)	Reference
ECG Electrodes (continued)			
High Demand ConMed Corp. Utica, NY	No	1.5	N/A
Holtrode ConMed Corp. Utica, NY	No	1.5	N/A
HP M2202A Radio-lucent Monitoring Electrode Ag/AgCL Hewlett-Packard Medical Supplies Andover, MA	No	1.5	N/A
Invisatrace Adult ECG Electrode ConMed Corp. Utica, NY	No	1.5	N/A
Pediatric Foam ConMed Corp. Utica, NY	No	1.5	N/A
Plia-Cell ConMed Corp. Utica, NY	No	1.5	N/A
Plia-Cell Diagnostic ConMed Corp. Utica, NY	No	1.5	N/A
Plia-Cell Diaphoretic ConMed Corp. Utica, NY	No	1.5	N/A
Quadtrode MRI ECG Electrode InVivo Research, Inc. Orlando, FL	No	1.5	N/A
Silvon ConMed Corp. Utica, NY	No	1.5	N/A
Silvon Adult ECG Electrode ConMed Corp. Utica, NY	No	1.5	N/A

Implant, material, device, or object	Attraction/ deflection	Highest field strength (T)	Reference
Silvon Diaphoretic ConMed Corp. Utica, NY	No	1.5	N/A
Silvon Stress ConMed Corp. Utica, NY	No	1.5	N/A
Snaptrace ConMed Corp. Utica, NY	No	1.5	N/A
SSE ConMed Corp. Utica, NY	No	1.5	N/A
SSE Radiotransparent ECG Electrode ConMed Corp. Utica, NY	No	1.5	N/A

Foley catheters with temperature sensors

Bardex I.C. Foley Catheter with silver and hydrogel coating, 16Fr. Bard Medical Division Covington, GA	No∞	1.5	N/A
Bardex Lubricath Temp. Sensing Urotrack Plus Foley Catheter with a 6 foot cable, 16 Fr. Bard Medical Division Covington, GA	No∞	1.5	N/A
Bardex I.C. Temp. Sensing Foley Catheter with a 6 foot cable, 16 Fr. Bard Medical Division Covington, GA	No∞	1.5	N/A

List of Items Tested

Implant, material, device, or object	Attraction/ deflection	Highest field strength (T)	Reference

Foley catheters with temperature sensors (continued)

Implant, material, device, or object	Attraction/ deflection	Highest field strength (T)	Reference
Bardex Pediatric Temp. Sensing 400-Series Urotrack Foley Catheter with a detachable cable, 12 Fr. Bard Medical Division Covington, GA	Yes∞	1.5	N/A
Extension cable for Foley Catheter with temperature sensor, 10 feet RSP Respiratory Support Products, Inc. SIMS Smiths Industries Irvine, CA	Yes∞	1.5	N/A
Foley Catheter with temperature sensor, 10 Fr. RSP Respiratory Support Products, Inc. SIMS Smiths Industries Irvine, CA	No∞	1.5	N/A
Foley Catheter with temperature sensor, 18 Fr. RSP Respiratory Support Products, Inc. SIMS Smiths Industries Irvine, CA	No∞	1.5	N/A

Halo vests and cervical fixation devices

Implant, material, device, or object	Attraction/ deflection	Highest field strength (T)	Reference
Ambulatory Halo System AOA Co. Greenwood, SC	Yes[a]	1.5	14

List of Items Tested

Implant, material, device, or object	Attraction/ deflection	Highest field strength (T)	Reference
Bremer standard halo crown and vest Bremmer Medical Co. Jacksonville, FL	No	1.0	15
Bremmer halo system MR-compatible Bremmer Medical Co. Jacksonville, FL	No	1.0	15
Closed-back halo (titanium) DePuy ACE Medical Co. El Segundo, CA	No	1.5	16
EXO adjustable coller Florida Manufacturing Co. Daytona, FL	Yes[a]	1.0	15
Guilford cervical orthosis Guilford & Son, Ltd. Cleveland, OH	Yes[a]	1.0	15
Guilford cervical orthosis, modified Guilford & Son, Ltd. Cleveland, OH	No	1.0	15
Mark III halo vest (aluminum superstructure, stainless steel rivets, titanium bolts) DePuy ACE Medical Co. El Segundo, CA	No	1.5	16
Mark IV halo vest (aluminum superstructure and titanium bolts) DePuy ACE Medical Co. El Segundo, CA	No	1.5	16
MR-compatible halo vest and cervical orthosis Lerman & Son Co. Beverly Hills, CA	No	1.5	N/A
Open-back halo (aluminum) DePuy ACE Medical Co. El Segundo, CA	No	1.5	16

List of Items Tested

Implant, material, device, or object	Attraction/ deflection	Highest field strength (T)	Reference
Halo vests and cervical fixation devices (continued)			
Open-back halo with Delrin inserts for skull pins (aluminum and Delrin) DePuy ACE Medical Co. El Segundo, CA	No	1.5	16
Philadelphia coller Philadelphia Coller Co. Westville, NJ	No	1.0	15
PMT halo cervical orthosis PMT Corp. Chanhassen, MN	No	1.0	15
PMT halo cervical orthosis with graphite rods and halo rings PMT Corp. Chanhassen, MN	No	1.0	15
S.O.M.I. cervical orthosis U.S. Manufacturing Co. Pasadena, CA	Yes[a]	1.0	15
Trippi-Wells tong (titanium) DePuy ACE Medical Co. El Segundo, CA	No	1.5	16
Heart valve prostheses			
Beall Coratomic Inc. Indiana, PA	Yes*	2.35	17
Bileaflet Model A7760 29 mm Medtronic Heart Valve Division Minneapolis, MN	No	1.5	N/A
Bjork-Shiley (convexo/concave) Shiley Inc. Irvine, CA	No	1.5	3
Bjork-Shiley (universal/spherical) Shiley Inc. Irvine, CA	Yes*	1.5	3

Implant, material, device, or object	Attraction/ deflection	Highest field strength (T)	Reference
Bjork-Shiley, Model MBC Shiley Inc. Irvine, CA	Yes*	2.35	19
Bjork-Shiley, Model 22 MBRC 11030 Shiley Inc. Irvine, CA	Yes*	2.35	19
CarboMedics Heart Valve Prosthesis Annuloflo Annuloplasty Ring Size 26 Carbomedics Austin, TX	No	1.5	N/A
CarboMedics Heart Valve Prosthesis Annuloflo Annuloplasty Ring Size 36 Carbomedics Austin, TX	No	1.5	N/A
CarboMedics Heart Valve Prosthesis Aortic Reduced, Model R500 Size 19 CarboMedics Austin, TX	No	1.5	18
CarboMedics Heart Valve Prosthesis Aortic Reduced, Model R500 Size 21 CarboMedics Austin, TX	No	1.5	18
CarboMedics Heart Valve Prosthesis Aortic Reduced, Model R500 Size 23 CarboMedics Austin, TX	No	1.5	18

Heart valve prostheses (continued)

Implant, material, device, or object	Attraction/ deflection	Highest field strength (T)	Reference
CarboMedics Heart Valve Prosthesis Aortic Reduced, Model R500 Size 25 CarboMedics Austin, TX	No	1.5	18
CarboMedics Heart Valve Prosthesis Aortic Reduced, Model R500 Size 27 CarboMedics Austin, TX	No	1.5	18
CarboMedics Heart Valve Prosthesis Aortic Reduced, Model R500 Size 29 CarboMedics Austin, TX	No	1.5	18
CarboMedics Heart Valve Prosthesis Aortic Standard, Model 500 Size 31 CarboMedics Austin, TX	No	1.5	18
CarboMedics Heart Valve Prosthesis Aortic Valve Size 16 Carbomedics Austin, TX	No	1.5	N/A
Carbomedics Heart Valve Prosthesis Carboseal Size 31 Carbomedics Austin, TX	No	1.5	N/A
CarboMedics Heart Valve Prosthesis Mitral Standard, Model 700	No	1.5	18

List of Items Tested

Implant, material, device, or object	Attraction/ deflection	Highest field strength (T)	Reference
Size 23 CarboMedics Austin, TX CarboMedics Heart Valve Prosthesis Mitral Standard, Model 700	No	1.5	18
Size 25 CarboMedics Austin, TX CarboMedics Heart Valve Prosthesis Mitral Standard, Model 700	No	1.5	18
Size 27 CarboMedics Austin, TX CarboMedics Heart Valve Prosthesis Mitral Standard, Model 700	No	1.5	18
Size 29 CarboMedics Austin, TX CarboMedics Heart Valve Prosthesis Mitral Standard, Model 700	No	1.5	18
Size 31 CarboMedics Austin, TX CarboMedics Heart Valve Prosthesis Mitral Standard, Model 700	No	1.5	18
Size 33 CarboMedics Austin, TX CarboMedics Heart Valve Prosthesis Mitral Valve Size 33 Carbomedics Austin, TX	No	1.5	N/A

Heart valve prostheses (continued)

Implant, material, device, or object	Attraction/ deflection	Highest field strength (T)	Reference
Carpentier-Edwards Annuloplasty Ring, Model 4400 Baxter Healthcare Corporation Santa Ana, CA	No	1.5	N/A
Carpentier-Edwards Annuloplasty Ring, Model 4500 Baxter Healthcare Corporation Santa Ana, CA	No	1.5	N/A
Carpentier-Edwards Annuloplasty Ring, Model 4600 Baxter Healthcare Corporation Santa Ana, CA	No	1.5	N/A
Carpentier-Edwards Bioprosthesis, Model 2625 Baxter Healthcare Corporation Santa Ana, CA	No	1.5	N/A
Carpentier-Edwards Bioprosthesis, Model 6625 Baxter Healthcare Corporation Santa Ana, CA	No	1.5	N/A
Carpentier-Edwards, Model 2650 American Edwards Laboratories Santa Ana, CA	Yes*	2.35	19
Carpentier-Edwards (porcine) American Edwards Laboratories Baxter Healthcare Corporation Santa Ana, CA	Yes*	2.35	19
Carpentier-Edwards Pericardial Bioprosthesis, Model 2700 Baxter Healthcare Corporation Santa Ana, CA	No	1.5	N/A
Carpentier-Edwards Physio Annuloplasty Ring, Model 4450	No	1.5	N/A

Implant, material, device, or object	Attraction/deflection	Highest field strength (T)	Reference
Baxter Healthcare Corporation Santa Ana, CA Cosgrove-Edwards Annuloplasty Ring, Model 4600	No	1.5	N/A
Baxter Healthcare Corporation Santa Ana, CA Duraflex Low Pressure Bioprosthesis, Model 6625E6R-LP	No	1.5	N/A
Baxter Healthcare Corporation Santa Ana, CA Duraflex Low Pressure Bioprosthesis, Model 6625LP	No	1.5	N/A
Baxter Healthcare Corporation Santa Ana, CA Duran Annuloplasty Ring Model H601H 35 mm Medtronic Heart Valve Division Minneapolis, MN	No	1.5	N/A
Freestyle Model 995 27 mm Medtronic Heart Valve Division Minneapolis, MN	No	1.5	N/A
Edwards-Duromedics Bileaflet Valve, Model 3160 Baxter Healthcare Corporation Santa Ana, CA	No	1.5	N/A
Edwards-Duromedics Bileaflet Valve, Model 9120 Baxter Healthcare Corporation Santa Ana, CA	No	1.5	N/A

Heart valve prostheses (continued)

Implant, material, device, or object	Attraction/ deflection	Highest field strength (T)	Reference
Edwards TEKNA Bileaflet Valve, Model 3200 Baxter Healthcare Corporation Santa Ana, CA	No	1.5	N/A
Edwards TEKNA Bileaflet Valve, Model 9200 Baxter Healthcare Corporation Santa Ana, CA	No	1.5	N/A
Hall-Kaster, Model A7700 Medtronic Minneapolis, MN	Yes*	1.5	3
Hancock 342 Model 342 35 mm Medtronic Heart Valve Division Minneapolis, MN	No	1.5	N/A
Hancock I (porcine) Johnson & Johnson Anaheim, CA	Yes*	1.5	3
Hancock II (porcine) Johnson & Johnson Anaheim, CA	Yes*	1.5	3
Hancock II Model T510 33 mm Medtronic Heart Valve Division Minneapolis, MN	No	1.5	N/A
Hancock Conduit Model 100 30 mm Medtronic Heart Valve Division Minneapolis, MN	No	1.5	N/A
Hancock extracorporeal Model 242R Johnson & Johnson Anaheim, CA	Yes*	2.35	18
Hancock extracorporeal Model M 4365-33	Yes*	2.35	18

List of Items Tested

Implant, material, device, or object	Attraction/ deflection	Highest field strength (T)	Reference
Johnson & Johnson Anaheim, CA Hancock Vascor, Model 505	No	2.35	19
Johnson & Johnson Anaheim, CA Inonescu-Shiley, Universal ISM	Yes*	2.35	19
Lillehi-Kaster, Model 300S Medical Inc. Inver Grove Heights, MN	Yes*	2.35	17
Lillehi-Kaster, Model 5009 Medical Inc. Inver Grove Heights, MN	Yes*	2.35	19

Med Hall Conduit
  Model R7700
  33 mm
Medtronic
Heart Valve Division
Minneapolis, MN
	No	1.5	N/A

Medtronic Hall Medtronic Inc. Minneapolis, MN	Yes*	2.35	18

Medtronic Hall
  Model 7700
  33 mm
Medtronic
Heart Valve Division
Minneapolis, MN
	No	1.5	N/A

Medtronic Hall Model A7700-D-16 Medtronic Inc. Minneapolis, MN	Yes*	2.35	18

Mosaic
  Model 310
  33 mm
Medtronic
Heart Valve Division
Minneapolis, MN
	No	1.5	N/A

Omnicarbon, Model 35231029 Medical Inc. Inver Grove Heights, MN	Yes*	2.35	18

Heart valve prostheses (continued)

Implant, material, device, or object	Attraction/ deflection	Highest field strength (T)	Reference
Omniscience, Model 6522 Medical Inc. Inver Grove Heights, MN	Yes*	2.35	18
On-X Valve, 6816 Medical Carbon Research Institute Austin, TX	No	1.5	N/A
Sculptor Annuloplasty Ring Model 605M 35 mm Medtronic Heart Valve Division Minneapolis, MN	No	1.5	N/A
Smeloff-Cutter Cutter Laboratories Berkeley, CA	Yes*	2.35	18
Sorin, No. 23	Yes*	1.5	20
Starr-Edwards, Model 1000 Baxter Healthcare Corporation Santa Ana, CA	Yes*	1.5	N/A
Starr-Edwards, Model 1200 Baxter Healthcare Corporation Santa Ana, CA	Yes*	1.5	N/A
Starr-Edwards, Model 1260 American Edwards Laboratories Baxter Healthcare Corporation Santa Ana, CA	Yes*	2.35	17
Starr-Edwards, Model 2300 Baxter Healthcare Corporation Santa Ana, CA	Yes*	1.5	N/A
Starr-Edwards, Model 2310 Baxter Healthcare Corporation Santa Ana, CA	Yes*	1.5	N/A
Starr-Edwards, Model 2320 American Edwards Laboratories Baxter Healthcare Corporation Santa Ana, CA	Yes*	2.35	17

List of Items Tested

Implant, material, device, or object	Attraction/ deflection	Highest field strength (T)	Reference
Starr-Edwards, Model 2400 American Edwards Laboratories Baxter Healthcare Corporation Santa Ana, CA	No	1.5	3
Starr-Edwards, Model Pre 6000 American Edwards Laboratories Baxter Healthcare Corporation Santa Ana, CA	Yes*	2.35	17
Starr-Edwards, Model 6000 Baxter Healthcare Corporation Santa Ana, CA	Yes*	1.5	N/A
Starr-Edwards, Model 6120 Baxter Healthcare Corporation Santa Ana, CA	Yes*	1.5	N/A
Starr-Edwards, Model 6300 Baxter Healthcare Corporation Santa Ana, CA	Yes*	1.5	N/A
Starr-Edwards, Model 6310 Baxter Healthcare Corporation Santa Ana, CA	Yes*	1.5	N/A
Starr-Edwards, Model 6320 Baxter Healthcare Corporation Santa Ana, CA	Yes*	1.5	N/A
Starr-Edwards, Model 6400 Baxter Healthcare Corporation Santa Ana, CA	Yes*	1.5	N/A
Starr-Edwards, Model 6520 Baxter Healthcare Corporation Santa Ana, CA	Yes*	2.35	19
St. Jude St. Jude Medical Inc. St. Paul, MN	No	1.5	3
St. Jude, Model A 101 St. Jude Medical Inc. St. Paul, MN	Yes*	2.35	19
St. Jude, Model M 101 St. Jude Medical Inc. St. Paul, MN	Yes*	2.35	19

List of Items Tested

Implant, material, device, or object	Attraction/ deflection	Highest field strength (T)	Reference
Intravascular coils, filters, and stents			
Amplatz IVC filter Cook, Inc. Bloomington, IN	No	4.7	21
AneuRX Graft Stent Medtronic AneuRx Sunnyvale, CA	No	1.5	N/A
Angiomed Memotherm Iliac 8 mm × 20 mm (Nitinol) C.R. Bard, Inc. Billerica, MA	No	1.5	N/A
Angiomed Memotherm Iliac 12 mm × 110 mm (Nitinol) C.R. Bard, Inc. Billerica, MA	No	1.5	N/A
Angiomed Memotherm Femoral 5 mm × 20 mm (Nitinol) C.R. Bard, Inc. Billerica, MA	No	1.5	N/A
Angiomed Memotherm Femoral 4 mm × 120 mm (Nitinol) C.R. Bard, Inc. Billerica, MA	No	1.5	N/A
AngioStent 15 mm (platinum, iridium) Angiodynamics Queensbury, NY	No	1.5	N/A
AngioStent	No	1.5	N/A
Cook occluding spring embolization coil, MWCE- 338-5-10	Yes*†	1.5	N/A
Cook-Z Stent Gianturco-Rosch Biliary Design 10 mm × 3 cm Cook, Inc. Bloomington, IN	Yes*†	1.5	N/A
Cook-Z Stent	Yes*†	1.5	N/A

List of Items Tested

Implant, material, device, or object	Attraction/ deflection	Highest field strength (T)	Reference
Gianturco-Rosch Tracheobronchial Design 20 mm × 5 cm Cook, Inc. Bloomington, IN			
Corvita Endoluminal Graft for Abdominal Aortic Aneurysm 27 × 120 Schneider (USA) Inc. Pfizer Medical Technology Group Minneapolis, MN	No	1.5	65
Cragg Nitinol spiral filter	No	4.7	21
Flower embolization microcoil (platinum) Target Therapeutics San Jose, CA	No	1.5	22
Gianturco embolization coil Cook, Inc. Bloomington, IN	Yes*†	1.5	21
Gianturco bird nest IVC filter Cook, Inc. Bloomington, IN	Yes*†	1.5	21, 23
Gianturco zig-zag stent Cook, Inc. Bloomington, IN	Yes*†	1.5	21
Greenfield vena cava filter (SS) MD Tech Watertown, MA	Yes*†	1.5	21, 24
Greenfield vena cava filter (titanium alloy) Ormco Glendora, CA	No	1.5	21
Guglielmi detachable coil (platinum) Target Therapeutics San Jose, CA	No	1.5	25
Gunther IVC filter William Cook, Europe	Yes*†	1.5	21

List of Items Tested

Implant, material, device, or object	Attraction/ deflection	Highest field strength (T)	Reference

Intravascular coils, filters, and stents (continued)

Implant, material, device, or object	Attraction/ deflection	Highest field strength (T)	Reference
Hilal embolization microcoil Cook, Inc. Bloomington, IN	No	1.5	23
Iliac Wallgraft Endoprosthesis 12 × 90 Schneider (USA) Inc. Pfizer Medical Technology Group Minneapolis, MN	No	1.5	65
Iliac Wallstent Endoprosthesis 5 × 80 Schneider (USA) Inc. Pfizer Medical Technology Group Minneapolis, MN	No	1.5	65
Iliac Wallstent Endoprosthesis Schneider (USA) Inc. 6 × 90 Pfizer Medical Technology Group Minneapolis, MN	No	1.5	65
Iliac Wallstent Endoprosthesis 12 × 90 Schneider (USA) Inc. Pfizer Medical Technology Group Minneapolis, MN	No	1.5	65
IVC venous clip (Teflon) Pilling Weck Co.	No	1.5	N/A
LGM IVC filter (Phynox) B. Braun Vena Tech Evanston, IL	No	1.5	26
Maas helical IVC filter Medinvent Lausanne, Switzerland	No	4.7	21

List of Items Tested

Implant, material, device, or object	Attraction/ deflection	Highest field strength (T)	Reference
Maas helical endovascular stent Medinvent Lausanne, Switzerland	No	4.7	21
Mobin-Uddin IVC/umbrella filter American Edwards Santa Ana, CA	No	4.7	21
MReye Embolization Coil William Cook A/S Bjaeverskov, Denmark	No	1.5	N/A
New retrievable IVC filter Thomas Jefferson University Philadelphia, PA	Yes*†	1.5	21
Palmaz endovascular stent Johnson & Johnson Interventional Warren, NJ	No	1.5	N/A
Palmaz endovascular stent Ethicon	Yes*†	1.5	21
Palmaz–Shatz balloon-expandable stent Johnson & Johnson Interventional Warren, NJ	Yes*†	1.5	N/A
Passager Stent (tantalum) 4 mm × 30 mm Meadox Surgimed Oakland, NJ	No	1.5	N/A
Passager Stent (tantalum) 10 mm × 30 mm Meadox Surgimed Oakland, NJ	No	1.5	N/A
Strecker stent (tantalum) MD Tech Watertown, MA	No	1.5	27
Talent Graft Stent bare spring model 8 × 16 mm (Nitinol) World Medical Manufacturing Corp. Sunrise, FL	No	1.5	N/A

List of Items Tested

Implant, material, device, or object	Attraction/ deflection	Highest field strength (T)	Reference

Intravascular coils, filters, and stents (continued)

Implant, material, device, or object	Attraction/ deflection	Highest field strength (T)	Reference
Talent Graft Stent open web model 8 × 16 mm (Nitinol) World Medical Manufacturing Corp. Sunrise, FL	No	1.5	N/A
Talent Graft Stent bare spring model 20 × 36 mm (Nitinol) World Medical Manufacturing Corp. Sunrise, FL	No	1.5	N/A
Talent Graft Stent open web model 20 × 36 mm (Nitinol) World Medical Manufacturing Corp. Sunrise, FL	No	1.5	N/A
Tracheobronchial Wallstent Endoprosthesis 14 × 80 Schneider (USA) Inc. Pfizer Medical Technology Group Minneapolis, MN	No	1.5	65
Tracheobronchial Wallstent Endoprosthesis 24 × 70 Schneider (USA) Inc. Pfizer Medical Technology Group Minneapolis, MN	No	1.5	65
Wallstent biliary endoprosthesis (high nickle stainless steel) Schneider USA Plymouth, MN	No	1.5	28

Implant, material, device, or object	Attraction/ deflection	Highest field strength (T)	Reference
Wallstent Endoprosthesis, Magic Wallstent 3.5 × 25 Schneider (USA) Inc. Pfizer Medical Technology Group Minneapolis, MN	No	1.5	65
Wallstent Endoprosthesis With Permalume covering 8 × 80 Schneider (USA) Inc. Pfizer Medical Technology Group Minneapolis, MN	No	1.5	65
Wallstent Esophageal II Endoprosthesis 20 × 130 Schneider (USA) Inc. Pfizer Medical Technology Group Minneapolis, MN	No	1.5	65
Wiktor coronary artery stent Medtronic Inverventional Vascular, Inc.	No	1.5	N/A
X-Trode, 3 segment (316 SS) C.R. Bard, Inc. Billerica, MA	No	1.5	N/A
X-Trode, 9 segment (316 SS) C.R. Bard, Inc. Billerica, MA	No	1.5	N/A
Ureteral stent	No	1.5	N/A

Ocular implants and devices

Implant, material, device, or object	Attraction/ deflection	Highest field strength (T)	Reference
Clip 50, double tantalum clip (tantalum) Mira Inc.	No	1.5	29
Clip 51, single tantalum clip (tantalum) Mira Inc.	No	1.5	29

Ocular implants and devices (continued)

Implant, material, device, or object	Attraction/ deflection	Highest field strength (T)	Reference
Clip 52, single tantalum clip (tantalum) Mira Inc.	No	1.5	29
Clip 250, double tantalum clip (tantalum) Mira Inc.	No	1.5	29
Double tantalum clip (tantalum) Storz Instrument Co.	No	1.5	29
Double tantalum clip style 250 (tantalum) Storz Instrument Co.	No	1.5	29
Fatio eyelid spring/wire	Yes	1.5	30
Gold eyelid spring	No	1.5	N/A
Intraocular lens implant Binkhorst, iridocapsular lense, platinum-iridium loop	No	1.5	31
Intraocular lens implant Binkhorst, iridocapsular lense, platinum-iridium loop (platinum, iridium)	No	1.0	31
Intraocular lens implant Binkhorst, iridocapsular lense, titanium loop (titanium)	No	1.0	31
Intraocular lens implant Worst, platinum clip lense	No	1.0	31
Retinal tack (303 SS) Bascom Palmer Eye Institute	No	1.5	32
Retinal tack (titanium alloy) Coopervision Irvine, CA	No	1.5	32
Retinal tack (303 SS) Duke	No	1.5	32
Retinal tack (cobalt, nickel) Greishaber Fallsington, PA	No	1.5	32
Retinal tack, Norton staple (platinum, rhodium) Norton	No	1.5	32

Implant, material, device, or object	Attraction/ deflection	Highest field strength (T)	Reference
Retinal tack (aluminum textraoxide) Ruby	No	1.5	32
Retinal tack (martensitic SS) Western European	Yes	1.5	32
Single tantalum clip (tantalum)	No	1.5	29
Troutman magnetic ocular implant	Yes	1.5	N/A
Unitech round wire eye spring	Yes	1.5	N/A

Orthopedic implants, materials, and devices

Implant, material, device, or object	Attraction/ deflection	Highest field strength (T)	Reference
AML femoral component bipolar hip prosthesis Zimmer Warsaw, IN	No	1.5	3
Cannulated cancellous screw 6.5 × 50 mm (titanium alloy) DePuy ACE Medical Co. El Segundo, CA	No	1.5	N/A
Captured screw assembly 100 mm (titanium alloy) DePuy ACE Medical Co. El Segundo, CA	No	1.5	N/A
Cervical wire, 18 gauge (316L SS)	No	0.3	33
Charnley-Muller hip prosthesis (Protasyl-10 alloy)	No	0.3	N/A
Cortical bone screw 4.5 × 36 mm (titanium alloy) DePuy ACE Medical Co. El Segundo, CA	No	1.5	N/A
Cortical bone screw, large (titanium alloy) Zimmer Warsaw, IN	No	1.5	34
Cortical bone screw, small (titanium alloy) Zimmer Warsaw, IN	No	1.5	34
Cotrel rods with hooks (316L SS)	No	0.3	33

Implant, material, device, or object	Attraction/ deflection	Highest field strength (T)	Reference

Orthopedic implants, materials, and devices (continued)

Cotrel rod (SS-ASTM, grade 2)	No	1.5	N/A
DTT, device for transverse traction (316L SS)	No	0.3	33
Drummond wire (316L SS)	No	0.3	33
Endoscopic noncannulated interference screw (titanium) Acufex Microsurgical Norwood, MA	No	1.5	34
Fixation staple (cobalt–chromium alloy) Richards Medical Co. Memphis, TN	No	1.5	34
Halifax clamps American Medical Electronics Richardson, TX	No	1.5	N/A
Harrington compression rod with hooks and nuts (316L SS)	No	0.3	33
Harrington distraction rod with hooks (316L SS)	No	0.3	33
Harris hip prosthesis Zimmer Warsaw, IN	No	1.5	3
Hip implant (austenitic SS) DePuy Inc. Warsaw, IN	No	1.5	N/A
Jewett nail Zimmer Warsaw, IN	No	1.5	3
Kirschner intermedullary rod Kirschner Medical Timonium, MD	No	1.5	3
"L" plate, 6-hole (titanium alloy) DePuy ACE Medical Co. El Segundo, CA	No	1.5	N/A
"L" Rod (cobalt–nickel alloy) Richards Medical Co. Memphis, TN	No	1.5	N/A
Luque Wire	No	0.3	33

List of Items Tested

Implant, material, device, or object	Attraction/deflection	Highest field strength (T)	Reference
Moe spinal instrumentation Zimmer Warsaw, IN	No	1.5	N/A
Perfix interence screw (17-4 SS) Instrument Makar Okemos, MI	Yes*	1.5	34
Rusch Rod	No	1.5	N/A
Side plate, 6-hole (titanium alloy) DePuy ACE Co. El Segundo, CA	No	1.5	N/A
Spinal L-Rod DePuy Warsaw, IN	No	1.5	N/A
Stainless steel plate Zimmer Warsaw, IN	No	1.5	3
Stainless steel screw Zimmer Warsaw, IN	No	1.5	3
Staple plate, large (Zimaloy) Zimmer Warsaw, IN	No	1.5	3
Stainless steel mesh Zimmer Warsaw, IN	No	1.5	3
Stainless steel wire Zimmer Warsaw, IN	No	1.5	3
Synthes AO DCP 2, 3, 4, 5 hole plate	No	1.5	N/A
Tibial nail, 9 mm (titanium alloy) DePuy ACE Medical Co. El Segundo, CA	No	1.5	N/A
Universal Reconstruction Ribbon (titanium) DePuy ACE Medical Co. El Segundo, CA	No	1.5	N/A
Zielke rod with screw, washer and nut (316L SS)	No	0.3	33

Otologic implants

Implant, material, device, or object	Attraction/ deflection	Highest field strength (T)	Reference
Austin tytan piston (titanium) Treace Medical Nashville, TN	No	1.5	35
Berger "V" bobbin ventilation tube (titanium) Richards Medical Co. Memphis, TN	No	1.5	35
Causse Flex H/A, notched, offset, partial ossicular prosthesis (titanium) Microtek Medical, Inc. Memphis, TN	No	1.5	36
Causse Flex H/A, notched, offset, total ossicular prosthesis (titanium) Microtek Medical Inc. Memphis, TN	No	1.5	36
Cochlear implant 3M/House	Yes	0.6	37
Cochlear implant 3M/Vienna	Yes	0.6	37
Cochlear implant Nucleus Mini 20-channel Cochlear Corporation Engelwood, CO	Yes	1.5	38
Cochlear implant, Combi 40/40+ Multichannel system MedEl Innsbrook, Austria	Yes∞	0.2 and 1.5	66, 67
Cody tack	No	0.6	37
Ehmke hook stapes prosthesis (platinum) Richards Medical Co. Memphis, TN	No	1.5	35
Flex H/A notched offset total ossicular prosthesis (316L SS)	No	1.5	36

Implant, material, device, or object	Attraction/ deflection	Highest field strength (T)	Reference
Microtek Medical, Inc. Memphis, TN			
Flex H/A offset partial ossicular prosthesis (316L SS)	No	1.5	36
Microtek Medical, Inc. Memphis, TN			
Fisch piston (Teflon, SS)	No	1.5	38
Richards Medical Co. Memphis, TN			
House single loop (ASTM-318-76, Grade 2 SS)	No	1.5	31
Storz St. Louis, MO			
House single loop (tantalum)	No	1.5	35
Storz St. Louis, MO			
House double loop (tantalum)	No	1.5	35
Storz St. Louis, MO			
House double loop (ASTM-318-76 Grade 2 SS)	No	1.5	35
Storz St. Louis, MO			
House-type incus prosthesis	No	0.6	N/A
House-type wire loop stapes prosthesis (316L SS)	No	1.5	35, 38
Richards Medical Co. Memphis, TN			
House-type stainless steel piston and wire (ASTM-318-76 Grade 2 SS)	No	1.5	35
Xomed-Treace Inc. A Bristol-Myers Squibb Co.			
House wire (tantalum)	No	0.5	39
Otomed			
House wire (SS)	No	0.5	39
Otomed			
McGee piston stapes prosthesis (316L, SS)	No	1.5	35, 38
Richards Medical Co. Memphis, TN			

Otologic implants (continued)

Implant, material, device, or object	Attraction/ deflection	Highest field strength (T)	Reference
McGee piston stapes prosthesis (platinum, 316L SS) Richards Medical Co. Memphis, TN	No	1.5	35, 38
McGee piston stapes prosthesis (platinum, chromium–nickel alloy, SS) Richards Medical Co. Memphis, TN	Yes	1.5	38
McGee Sheperd's Cook stapes prosthesis (316L SS) Richards Medical Co. Memphis, TN	No	1.5	35
Plasti-pore piston (316L SS/ Plasti-pore material) Richards Medical Co. Memphis, TN	No	1.5	35, 38
Platinum ribbon loop stapes prosthesis (platinum) Richards Medical Co. Memphis, TN	No	1.5	35
Reuter bobbin ventilation tube (316L SS) Richards Medical Co. Memphis, TN	No	1.5	35
Reuter drain tube	No	1.5	35
Richards bucket handle stapes prosthesis (316L SS) Richards Medical Co. Memphis, TN	No	1.5	35, 38
Richards Plasti-pore with Armstrong-style platinum ribbon (platinum) Richards Medical Co. Memphis, TN	No	1.5	35
Richards platinum Teflon piston, 0.6 mm (Teflon, platinum) Richards Medical Co. Memphis, TN	No	1.5	38

List of Items Tested

Implant, material, device, or object	Attraction/ deflection	Highest field strength (T)	Reference
Richards platinum Teflon piston, 0.8 mm (Teflon, platinum) Richards Medical Co. Memphis, TN	No	1.5	38
Richards piston stapes prosthesis (platinum, fluoroplastic) Richards Medical Co. Memphis, TN	No	1.5	35
Richards Shepherd's crook (platinum) Richards Medical Co. Memphis, TN	No	0.5	39
Richards Teflon piston (Teflon) Richards Medical Co. Memphis, TN	No	1.5	38
Robinson–Moon–Lippy offset stapes prosthesis (ASTM-318-76 Grade 2 SS) Storz St. Louis, MO	No	1.5	35
Robinson–Moon offset stapes prosthesis (ASTM-318-76 Grade 2 SS) Storz St. Louis, MO	No	1.5	35
Robinson incus replacement prosthesis (ASTM-318-76 Grade 2 SS) Storz St. Louis, MO	No	1.5	35
Robinson stapes prosthesis (ASTM-318-76 Grade 2 SS) Storz St. Louis, MO	No	1.5	35
Ronis piston stapes prosthesis (316L SS, fluoroplastic) Richards Medical Co. Memphis, TN	No	1.5	35

Otologic implants (continued)

Implant, material, device, or object	Attraction/ deflection	Highest field strength (T)	Reference
Schea cup piston stapes prosthesis (platinum, fluoroplastic) Richards Medical Co. Memphis, TN	No	1.5	35, 38
Schea malleus attachment piston (Teflon) Richards Medical Co. Memphis, TN	No	1.5	38
Schea stainless steel and Teflon wire prosthesis (Teflon, 316 L SS) Richards Medical Co. Memphis, TN	No	1.5	38
Scheer piston stapes prosthesis (316L SS, fluoroplastic) Richards Medical Co. Memphis, TN	No	1.5	35
Scheer piston (Teflon, 316L SS) Richards Medical Co. Memphis, TN	No	1.5	33
Schuknecht gelfoam and wire prosthesis, Armstrong style (316L SS) Richards Medical Co. Memphis, TN	No	1.5	40
Schuknecht piston stapes prosthesis (316L SS, fluoroplastic) Richards Medical Co. Memphis, TN	No	1.5	35
Schuknecht Tef-wire incus attachment (ASTM-318-76 Grade 2 SS) Storz St. Louis, MO	No	1.5	35, 38
Schuknecht Tef-wire malleus attachment (ASTM-318-76 Grade 2 SS) Storz St. Louis, MO	No	1.5	35, 38

List of Items Tested

Implant, material, device, or object	Attraction/ deflection	Highest field strength (T)	Reference
Schuknecht Teflon wire piston 0.6 mm (Teflon, 316L SS) Richards Medical Co. Memphis, TN	No	1.5	38
Schuknecht Teflon wire piston 0.8 mm (Teflon, 316L SS) Richards Medical Co. Memphis, TN	No	1.5	38
Sheehy incus replacement (ASTM-318-76 Grade 2 SS) Storz St. Louis, MO	No	1.5	35
Sheehy incus strut (316L SS) Richards Medical Co. Memphis, TN	No	1.5	38
Sheehy-type incus replacement strut (Teflon, 316L SS) Richards Medical Co. Memphis, TN	No	1.5	35
Silverstein malleus clip ventilation tube (Teflon, 316L SS) Richards Medical Co. Memphis, TN	No	1.5	38
Spoon bobbin ventilation tube (316L SS) Richards Medical Co. Memphis, TN	No	1.5	35
Stapes fluoroplastic/platinum piston Microtek Medical, Inc. Memphis, TN	No	1.5	36
Stapes fluoroplastic/stainless steel piston (316L SS) Microtek Medical, Inc. Memphis, TN	No	1.5	36
Tantalum wire loop stages prosthesis (tantalum) Richards Medical Co. Memphis, TN	No	1.5	35, 38

List of Items Tested

Implant, material, device, or object	Attraction/ deflection	Highest field strength (T)	Reference

Otologic implants (continued)

Implant, material, device, or object	Attraction/ deflection	Highest field strength (T)	Reference
Tef-platinum piston (platinum) Xomed-Treace Inc. A Bristol-Myers Squibb Co.	No	1.5	35
Total ossicular replacement prosthesis (TORP) (316L SS) Richards Medical Co. Memphis, TN	No	1.5	38
Trapeze ribbon loop stapes prosthesis (platinum) Richards Medical Co. Memphis, TN	No	1.5	35
Williams microclip (316L SS) Richards Medical Co. Memphis, TN	No	1.5	35
Xomed stapes (ASTM-318-76 Grade 2 SS) Xomed-Treace Inc. A Bristol-Myers Squibb Co.	No	1.5	35
Xomed ceravital partial ossicular prosthesis	No	1.5	N/A
Xomed Baily stapes implant	No	1.5	35
Xomed stapes prosthesis Robinson-style Richard's Co. Nashville, TN	No	1.5	35

Patent ductus arteriosus (PDA), atrial septal defect (ASD), and ventricular septal defect (VSD) occluders

Implant, material, device, or object	Attraction/ deflection	Highest field strength (T)	Reference
Rashkind PDA Occlusion Implant 12 mm, lot n. 071C1391 (304V SS) C.R. Bard, Inc. Billerica, MA	Yes[†]	1.5	41
Rashkind PDA Occlusion Implant 17 mm, lot no. 514486 (304 V SS) C.R. Bard, Inc. Billerica, MA	Yes[†]	1.5	41

List of Items Tested

Implant, material, device, or object	Attraction/ deflection	Highest field strength (T)	Reference
Lock Clamshell Septal Occlusion Implant 17 mm, lot no. 07BCO321 (304 V SS) C.R. Bard, Inc. Billerica, MA	Yes[†]	1.5	41
Lock Clamshell Septal Occlusion Implant 23 mm, lot no. 07CC1903 (304 V SS) C.R. Bard, Inc. Billerica, MA	Yes[†]	1.5	41
Lock Clamshell Septal Occlusion Implant 28 mm, lot no. 07BC1557 (304 V SS) C.R. Bard, Inc. Billerica, MA	Yes[†]	1.5	41
Lock Clamshell Septal Occlusion Implant 33 mm, lot no. 07AC1785 (304 V SS) C.R. Bard, Inc. Billerica, MA	Yes[†]	1.5	41
Lock Clamshell Septal Occlusion Implant 40 mm, lot no. 07AC1785 (304 V SS) C.R. Bard, Inc. Billerica, MA	Yes[†]	1.5	41
Bard Clamshell Septal Umbrella 17 mm, lot no. 09ED1230 (MP35N) C.R. Bard, Inc. Billerica, MA	No	1.5	41
Bard Clamshell Septal Umbrella 23 mm, lot no. 09ED1232 (MP35N) C.R. Bard, Inc. Billerica, MA	No	1.5	41

Patent ductus arteriosus (PDA), atrial septal defect (ASD), and ventricular septal defect (VSD) occluders (continued)

Implant, material, device, or object	Attraction/ deflection	Highest field strength (T)	Reference
Bard Clamshell Septal Umbrella 28 mm, lot no. 09ED1233 (MP35N) C.R. Bard, Inc. Billerica, MA	No	1.5	41
Bard Clamshell Septal Umbrella 33 mm, lot no. 09ED1234 (MP35N) C.R. Bard, Inc. Billerica, MA	No	1.5	41
Bard Clamshell Septal Umbrella 40 mm, lot no. 09ED1231 (MP35N) C.R. Bard, Inc. Bellerica, MA	No	1.5	41

Pellets and bullets

Implant, material, device, or object	Attraction/ deflection	Highest field strength (T)	Reference
BB's (Daisy)	Yes	1.5	N/A
BBs (Crosman)	Yes	1.5	N/A
Bullet, .380 inch (copper, plastic, lead) Glaser	No	1.5	42
Bullet, .44 inch (Teflon, bronze) North American Ordinance	No	1.5	42
Bullet, 7.62 × 39 mm (copper, steel) Norinco	Yes	1.5	42
Bullet, .357 inch (copper, lead) Cascade	No	1.5	42
Bullet, .357 inch (lead) Remington	No	1.5	42
Bullet, .357 inch (aluminum, lead) Winchester	No	1.5	42

Implant, material, device, or object	Attraction/ deflection	Highest field strength (T)	Reference
Bullet, 9 mm (copper, lead) Remington	No	1.5	42
Bullet, .380 inch (copper, nickel, lead) Winchester	Yes	1.5	42
Bullet, .357 inch (nylon, lead) Smith & Wesson	No	1.5	42
Bullet, .357 inch (nickel, copper, lead) Winchester	No	1.5	42
Bullet, .45 inch (steel, lead) Evansville Ordinance	Yes	1.5	42
Bullet, .357 inch (steel, lead) Fiocchi	No	1.5	42
Bullet, .357 inch (copper, lead) Hornady	No	1.5	42
Bullet, 9 mm (copper, lead) Norma	Yes	1.5	42
Bullet, .357 inch (bronze, plastic) Patton-Morgan	No	1.5	42
Bullet, .357 inch (copper, lead) Patton–Morgan	No	1.5	42
Bullet, .45 inch (copper, lead) Samson	No	1.5	42
Shot, 12 gauge, size: 00 (copper, lead) Federal	No	1.5	42
Shot, 7 1/2 (lead)	No	1.5	42
Shot, 4 (lead)	No	1.5	42
Shot, 00 buckshot (lead)	No	1.5	42

Penile implants

Implant, material, device, or object	Attraction/ deflection	Highest field strength (T)	Reference
Penile implant, AMS 700 CX Inflatable American Medical Systems Minnetonka, MN	No	1.5	43
Penile implant, AMS 700 CX/ CXM American Medical Systems Minnetonka, MN	No	1.5	N/A

Penile implants (continued)

Implant, material, device, or object	Attraction/ deflection	Highest field strength (T)	Reference
Penile implant, AMS 700 Ultrex American Medical Systems Minnetonka, MN	No	1.5	N/A
Penile implant, 700 Ultrex Plus American Medical Systems Minnetonka, MN	No	1.5	N/A
Penile implant, AMS Ambicor American Medical Systems Minnetonka, MN	No	1.5	N/A
Penile implant, AMS Dynaflex American Medical Systems Minnetonka, MN	No	1.5	N/A
Penile implant, AMS Hydroflex self-contained American Medical Systems Minnetonka, MN	No	1.5	N/A
Penile implant, AMS Malleable 600 American Medical Systems Minnetonka, MN	No	1.5	43
Penile implant, AMS Malleable 600M American Medical Systems Minnetonka, MN	No	1.5	N/A
Penile implant, AMS Malleable 650 American Medical Systems Minnetonka, MN	No	1.5	N/A
Penile implant, Duraphase	Yes	1.5	N/A
Penile implant, Flexi-Flate Surgitek Medical Engineering Corp. Racine, WI	No	1.5	43
Penile implant, Flexi-Rod (Standard) Surgitek Medical Engineering Corp. Racine, WI	No	1.5	43
Penile implant, Osmond, external	No	1.5	N/A

Implant, material, device, or object	Attraction/deflection	Highest field strength (T)	Reference
Penile implant, Flex-Rod II (Firm) Surgitek Medical Engineering Corp. Racine, WI	No	1.5	43
Penile implant, Jonas Dacomed Corp. Minneapolis, MN	No	1.5	43
Penile implant, Mentor Flexible Mentor Corp. Minneapolis, MN	No	1.5	43
Penile implant, Mentor Inflatable Mentor Corp. Minneapolis, MN	No	1.5	43
Penile implant, OmniPhase Dacomed Corp. Minneapolis, MN	Yes	1.5	43
Penile implant, Uniflex 1000	No	1.5	N/A

Vascular access ports and catheters

A Port Implantable Access System (titanium) Therex Corporation Walpole, MA	No	1.5	44
Access Implantable (titanium, plastic) Celsa Cedex, France	No	1.5	44
Broviac Catheter single lumen (silicone, barium sulfate) Bard Access Systems Salt Lake City, UT	No	1.5	45
Button (polysulfone polymer, silicone) Infusaid Inc. Norwood, MA	No	1.5	44
CathLink LP (titanium) Bard Access Systems Salt Lake City, UT	No	1.5	45

List of Items Tested

Implant, material, device, or object	Attraction/ deflection	Highest field strength (T)	Reference
Vascular access ports and catheters (continued)			
CathLink SP (titanium) Bard Access Systems Salt Lake City, UT	No	1.5	45
Celsite Port and Catheter (titanium) B. Braun Medical Bethlehem, PA	No	1.5	44
Dome Port (titanium) Davol Inc., Subsidiary of C.R. Bard, Inc. Cranston, RI	No	1.5	44
Dual MacroPort (polysulfone polymer, silicone) Infusaid Inc. Norwood, MA	No	1.5	44
Dual MicroPort (polysulfone polymer, silicone) Infusaid Inc. Norwood, MA	No	1.5	44
Groshong Catheter	Yes*	1.5	N/A
Groshong Catheter, dual lumen, 9.5 Fr. (silicone, barium sulfate, tungsten) Bard Access Systems Salt Lake City, UT	No	1.5	45
Groshong Catheter, single lumen, 8 Fr. (silicone, barium sulfate, tungsten) Bard Access Systems Salt Lake City, UT	No	1.5	45
Hickman Catheter, single lumen, 3.0 Fr. Bard Access Systems Salt Lake City, UT	No	1.5	45
Hickman Catheter, dual lumen, 10.0 Fr. (silicone, barium sulfate) Bard Access Systems Salt Lake City, UT	No	1.5	45

List of Items Tested

Implant, material, device, or object	Attraction/ deflection	Highest field strength (T)	Reference
Hickman Port (316L SS) Davol Inc., Subsidiary of C.R. Bard, Inc. Cranston, RI	Yes*	1.5	44
Hickman Port, Pediatric (titanium) Davol, Inc., Subsidiary of C.R. Bard, Inc. Salt Lake City, UT	No	1.5	44
Hickman subcutaneous port attachable venous catheter (titanium) Davol, Inc., Subsidiary of C.R. Bard, Inc. Salt Lake City, UT	No	1.5	45
Hickman subcutaneous port venous catheter preconnected (titanium) Davol Inc., Subsidiary of C.R. Bard, Inc. Salt Lake City, UT	No	1.5	44
Hickman subcutaneous port (SS, titanium, plastic) Davol, Inc., Subsidiary of C.R. Bard, Inc. Salt Lake City, UT	No	1.5	45
HMP-Port (plastic) Horizon Medical Products Atlanta, GA	No	1.5	44
Implantofix II (polysulfone) Burron Medical Inc. Bethlehem, PA	No	1.5	44
Infusaid, Model 400 (titanium) Infusaid Inc. Norwood, MA	No	1.5	44
Infusaid, Model 600 (titanium) Infusaid Inc. Norwood, MA	No	1.5	44
Infuse-A-Kit (plastic) Infusaid Norwood, MA	No	1.5	44

List of Items Tested

Implant, material, device, or object	Attraction/ deflection	Highest field strength (T)	Reference

Vascular access ports and catheters (continued)

Implant, material, device, or object	Attraction/ deflection	Highest field strength (T)	Reference
LifePort, Model 6013 (Delrin) Strato Medical Corporation Beverly, MA	No	1.5	44
Lifeport, Model 1013 (titanium) Strato Medical Corp. Beverly, MA	No	1.5	44
LifePort Vascular Access System attachable catheter (plastic) Strato Medical Group Beverly, MA	No	1.5	44
LifePort Vascular Access System attachable catheter and bayonet lock ring (plastic) Strato Medical Group Beverly, MA	No	1.5	44
Low Profile MRI Port (Delrin) Davol, Inc., Subsidiary of C.R. Bard, Inc. Salt Lake City, UT	No	1.5	45
Low Profile MRI Port (titanium) Davol, Inc. Subsidiary of C.R. Bard, Inc. Salt Lake City, UT	No	1.5	45
Macroport (polysulfone, titanium) Infusaid Inc. Norwood, MA	No	1.5	N/A
Mediport Cormed	No	1.5	N/A
MicroPort (polysulfone, polymersilicone) Infusaid Inc. Norwood, MA	No	1.5	44
MRI Dual Port (Delrin, titanium) Davol, Inc., Subsidiary of C.R. Bard, Inc. Salt Lake City, UT	No	1.5	45
MRI Hard Base Implanted Port (plastic)	No	1.5	44

Implant, material, device, or object	Attraction/ deflection	Highest field strength (T)	Reference
Davol, Inc., Subsidiary of C.R. Bard, Inc. Salt Lake City, UT			
MRI Port (Delrin, silicone) Davol, Inc., Subsidiary of C.R. Bard, Inc. Salt Lake City, UT	No	1.5	44
Norport-AC (titanium) Norfolk Medical Skokie, IL	No	1.5	44
Norport-DL (316L SS) Norfolk Medical Skokie, IL	No	1.5	44
Norport-LS (titanium) Norfolk Medical Skokie, IL	No	1.5	44
Norport-LS (316L SS) Norfolk Medical Skokie, IL	No	1.5	44
Norport-LS (polysulfone) Norfolk Medical Skokie, IL	No	1.5	44
Norport-PT (titanium) Norfolk Medical Skokie, IL	No	1.5	44
Norport-SP (polysulfone, silicone rubber, Dacron) Norfolk Medical Skokie, IL	No	1.5	44
OmegaPort Access System (titanium, 316L SS) Norfolk Medical Skokie, IL	No	1.5	44
OmegaPort-SR Access System (titanium, 316L SS) Norfolk Medical Skokie, IL	No	1.5	44
Open-ended Catheter, single lumen, 6 Fr. (ChronoFlex) Davol, Inc., Subsidiary of C.R. Bard, Inc. Salt Lake City, UT	No	1.5	45

List of Items Tested

Implant, material, device, or object	Attraction/ deflection	Highest field strength (T)	Reference

Vascular access ports and catheters (continued)

Implant, material, device, or object	Attraction/ deflection	Highest field strength (T)	Reference
Open-ended Catheter, single lumen, 8 Fr. (ChronoFlex) Davol, Inc., Subsidiary of C.R. Bard, Inc. Salt Lake City, UT	No	1.5	45
OptiPort Catheter, single lumen (silicone) Simms-Deltec St. Paul, MN	No	1.5	45
PeriPort (polysulfone, titanium) Infusaid, Inc. Norwood, MA	No	1.5	44
Phantom Norfolk Medical Skokie, IL	No	1.5	44
Plastic Port (polysulfone, titanium) Cardial Saint-Etienne, France	No	1.5	45
Port-A-Cath, P.S.A. Port Portal (titanium) Pharmacia Deltec St. Paul, MN	No	1.5	44
Port-A-Cath Titanium Dual Lumen Portal (titanium) Pharmacia Deltec St. Paul, MN	No	1.5	44
Port-A-Cath Titanium Peritoneal Portal (titanium) Pharmacia Deltec St. Paul, MN	No	1.5	44
Port-A-Cath Titanium Venous Low Profile Portal (titanium) Pharmacia Deltec St. Paul, MN	No	1.5	44
Port-A-Cath Titanium Venous Portal (titanium) Pharmacia Deltec St. Paul, MN	No	1.5	44

List of Items Tested

Implant, material, device, or object	Attraction/ deflection	Highest field strength (T)	Reference
Porto-cath Pharmacin, NUTECH Pharmacia Deltec St. Paul, MN	No	1.5	44
Q-Port (316L SS) Quinton Instrument Co. Seattle, WA	Yes*	1.5	44
R-Port Premier (silicone, plastic, SS) Medi-tech Boston Scientific Corp. Watertown, MA	No	1.5	N/A
S.E.A. (titanium) Harbor Medical Devices, Inc. Boston, MA	No	1.5	44
Snap-Lock (titanium, polysulfone polymer, silicone) Infusaid Inc. Norwood, MA	No	1.5	44
Synchromed, Model 8500-1 (titanium, thermoplastic, silicone) Medtronic, Inc. Minneapolis, MN	No	1.5	44
TitanPort (titanium) Norfolk Medical Skokie, IL	No	1.5	N/A
Triple Lumen Arrow International, Inc. Reading, PA	No	1.5	N/A
Vasport (titanium, fluoropolymer) Gish Biomedical, Inc. Santa Ana, CA	No	1.5	44
Vascular Access Catheter With Repair Kit PMT Corporation Chanhassen, MN	No	1.5	N/A

List of Items Tested

Implant, material, device, or object	Attraction/ deflection	Highest field strength (T)	Reference

Vascular access ports and catheters (continued)

Implant, material, device, or object	Attraction/ deflection	Highest field strength (T)	Reference
Vaxess, plastic (plastic, polyurethane) Medi-tech Boston Scientific Corp. Watertown, MA	No	1.5	N/A
Vaxess, titanium (titanium, polyurethane) Medi-tech Boston Scientific Corp. Watertown, MA	No	1.5	N/A
Vaxess, titanium mini-port with silicone catheter (titanium, silicone) Medi-tech Boston Scientific Corp. Watertown, MA	No	1.5	N/A
Vital-Port (polysulfone, titanium) Cook Pacemaker Corp. Leechburg, PA	No	1.5	45
Vital-Port, Dual (polysulfone, titanium) Cook Pacemaker Corp. Leechburg, PA	No	1.5	45

Miscellaneous

Implant, material, device, or object	Attraction/ deflection	Highest field strength (T)	Reference
0.22 Magnum Minirevolver North American Arms Spanish Fork, UT	Yes	1.5	46
0.380-caliber Semiautomatic Model BDA-380 Browing Morgan, UT	Yes	1.5	46
9-mm Semiautomatic Model PT-92C Taurus International Miami, FL	Yes	1.5	46

List of Items Tested

Implant, material, device, or object	Attraction/ deflection	Highest field strength (T)	Reference
357 Magnum Revolver Model 66-3 Smith and Wesson Springfield, MA	Yes	1.5	46
Accusite pH Enteral Feeding System pH Site Locator 10 Fr. Zinetics Medical Salt Lake City, UT	No[††††]	1.5	N/A
Adson Tissue Forcep (Ti6Al-4V) Johnson and Johnson Professional, Inc. Raynham, MA	No	1.5	63
Artificial urinary sphincter AMS 800 American Medical Systems Minnetonka, MN	No	1.5	3
AMS Artificial Bowel Sphincter Prosthesis American Medical Systems Minnetonka, MN	No	1.5	N/A
AMS Mainstay Soft-Tissue Anchor American Medical Systems Minnetonka, MN	No	1.5	N/A
AMS Artificial Urinary Sphincter 791 American Medical Systems Minnetonka, MN	No	1.5	N/A
Battery, lithium, 3.9 Volt (304 SS and 316L SS, nickle) Greatbatch Scientific Clarence, NY	Yes*	1.5	N/A
Biosearch endo-feeding tube	No	1.5	N/A
Cerebral ventricular shunt tube connector Accu-Flow, straight Codman Randolf, MA	No	1.5	3

Miscellaneous (continued)

Implant, material, device, or object	Attraction/ deflection	Highest field strength (T)	Reference
Cerebral ventricular shunt tube connector Accu-flow, right angle Codman Randolf, MA	No	1.5	3
Cerebral ventricular shunt tube connector Accu-flow, T-connector Codman Randolf, MA	No	1.5	3
Cerebral ventricular shunt tube connector (type unknown)	Yes	0.147	1
Codman-Medos Programmable Valve Medos S.A. LeLocle, Switzerland	Yes	1.5	68
Contraceptive diaphragm All Flex Ortho Pharmaceutical Raritan, NJ	Yes*	1.5	3
Contraceptive diaphragm Flat Spring Ortho Pharmaceutical Raritan, NJ	Yes*	1.5	3
Contraceptive diaphragm Gyne T	No	1.5	47
Contraceptive diaphragm Koroflex Young Drug Products Piscataway, NJ	Yes*	1.5	3
Contraceptive IUD Multiload CU375 (copper, silver)	No	1.5	47
Contraceptive IUD Nova T (copper, silver)	No	1.5	47
Cranial Ceramic Drill bit (ceramic) MicroSurgical Techniques Inc. Fort Collins, CO	No	1.5	48, 49

Implant, material, device, or object	Attraction/ deflection	Highest field strength (T)	Reference
Craniofix, bone flap fixation system (titanium alloy) Aesculap, Inc. South San Francisco, CA	No	1.5	50
CT-MRI Topographic Marker E-Z-Em Westbury, NY	No	1.5	N/A
Deponit, nitroglycerin transdermal delivery system (aluminized plastic) Schwarz Pharma Milwaukee, WI	No[†††]	1.5	N/A
EEG electrodes, Pediatric E-5-GH (gold plated silver) Grass Co. Quincy, MA	No	0.3	51
EEG electrodes, Adult E-6-GH (gold plated silver) Grass Co. Quincy, MA	No	0.3	51
Endotracheal tube with metal ring marker Trachmate	No	1.5	N/A
Endoscope, rigid, 8.0 mm (Laryngoscope) Greatbatch Scientific Clarence, NY	No	1.5	60
Endoscope, rigid, 2.7 mm (Sinuscope) Greatbatch Scientific Clarence, NY	No	1.5	60
Eyelid weight (gold)	No	1.5	52
Fiber-optic Intubating Laryngoscope Blade Greatbatch Scientific Clarence, NY	No	1.5	N/A
Fiber-optic Intubating Laryngoscope Handle Greatbatch Scientific Clarence, NY	No	1.5	N/A

Miscellaneous (continued)

Implant, material, device, or object	Attraction/ deflection	Highest field strength (T)	Reference
Firestar 9-mm semiautomatic Star Bonifacio Echeverria Eibar, Spain	Yes	1.5	46
Flex-tip Plus Epidural catheter (304V SS) Arrow International Inc. Reading, PA	Yes[††††]	1.5	N/A
Forceps (titanium)	No	1.39	1
Forceps (ceramic) MicroSurgical Techniques Inc. Fort Collins, CO	No	1.5	48, 49
Hakim valve and pump	No	1.39	1
Implantable Spinal Fusion Stimulator Electro-Biology, Inc. (EBI) Parsippany, NJ	Yes∞	1.5	64
Intracranial depth electrodes for EEG recordings (nickle-chromium alloy) Superior Tube Company Norristown, NY	No	1.5	53
Intraflex Feeding Tube tungstun weight, plastic	No	1.5	N/A
Intrauterine contraceptive device (IUD), Copper T (copper) Searle Pharmaceuticals Chicago, IL	No	1.5	54
Intrauterine contraceptive device (IUD), Lippey loop, plastic	No	1.5	N/A
Intrauterine contraceptive device (IUD) Perigard Gyne Pharmaceuticals	No	1.5	N/A

List of Items Tested

Implant, material, device, or object	Attraction/ deflection	Highest field strength (T)	Reference
Langenbeck Periosteal Elevator (304 SS) Johnson and Johnson Professional, Inc. Raynham, MA	No	1.5	63
Laparoscopic Graspers Greatbatch Scientific Clarence, NY	No	1.5	N/A
Low Magnetic Signature Lithium Battery (C size) Greatbatch Scientific Clarence, NY	No	1.5	N/A
May Hegar Needle Holder (titanium alloy) Johnson and Johnson Professional, Inc. Raynham, MA	No	1.5	63
Mercury Duotube-feeding	No	1.5	N/A
Micro Needle Holder Greatbatch Scientific Clarence, NY	No	1.5	N/A
Micro Tissue Forceps Greatbatch Scientific Clarence, NY	No	1.5	N/A
Micro Round Handled Scissors Greatbatch Scientific Clarence, NY	No	1.5	N/A
Micro Tying Forceps Greatbatch Scientific Clarence, NY	No	1.5	N/A
Mitek anchor	No	1.5	N/A
Penfield Dissector (304 SS) Johnson and Johnson Professional, Inc. Raynham, MA	No	1.5	63
Peripheral Nerve Stimulator MR-STIM, Model GN-013 Greatbatch Scientific Clarence, NY	No	1.5	N/A

List of Items Tested

Implant, material, device, or object	Attraction/ deflection	Highest field strength (T)	Reference
Miscellaneous (continued)			
Scalpel, Microsharp Ceramic Scalpels, sizes #10, #11, #11c, #15 (ceramic) MicroSurgical Techniques Inc. Fort Collins, CO	No	1.5	48, 49
Scalpel (SS)	Yes	1.5	N/A
Scissors, Ceramic (prototype) (ceramic) Microsurgical Techniques, Inc. Fort Collins, CO	No	1.5	48, 49
Shunt valve, Holtertype The Holter Co. Bridgeport, PA	Yes*	1.5	55
Shunt valve, Holter–Hausner type Holter–Hausner, Inc. Bridgeport, PA	No	1.5	55
Sophy adjustable pressure valve	Yes	1.5	56
Sophy programmable pressure valve Model SM8 Sophysa Orsay, France	Yes∞	1.5	68
Sophy programmable pressure valve Model SP3 Sophysa Orsay, France	Yes∞	1.5	68
Sophy programmable pressure valve Model SU8 Sophysa Orsay, France	Yes∞	1.5	68
Sponge Forcep (titanium alloy) Johnson and Johnson Professional, Inc. Raynham, MA	No	1.5	63

List of Items Tested

Implant, material, device, or object	Attraction/ deflection	Highest field strength (T)	Reference
Stereotactic headframe with removable mouthpiece (aluminum, 8–18 SS Delrin, titanium) Compass International, Inc. Rochester, MN	No	1.5	N/A
Suction/Irrigation Handle for Sinuscope Greatbatch Scientific Clarence, NY	No	1.5	N/A
SynchroMed, implantable drug infusion device Medtronic Inc.	No$^{\infty}$	1.5	N/A
Super ArrowFlex PSI 9 Fr. × 11 cm (304 V SS) Arrow International Inc. Reading, PA	Yes††††	1.5	N/A
Super ArrowFlex PSI 10 Fr. × 65 cm (304V SS) Arrow International Inc. Reading, PA	Yes††††	1.5	N/A
Tantalum powder	No	1.39	1
TheraCath (304 V SS) Arrow International Inc. Reading, PA	Yes††††	1.5	N/A
Tweezers, Ceramic (prototype) (ceramic) MicroSurgical Techniques, Inc. Fort Collins, CO	No	1.5	48, 48
Vascular marker, O-ring washer (302 SS) PIC Design, Middlebury, CT	Yes*	1.5	N/A
UroLume Endoprosthesis (titanium) American Medical Systems Minnetonka, MN	No	1.5	N/A
Vitallium implant	No	1.5	N/A

List of Items Tested

Implant, material, device, or object	Attraction/ deflection	Highest field strength (T)	Reference
Miscellaneous (continued)			

Winged infusion set
  MRI compatible
  E-Z-EM Inc.
  Westbury, NY
	No	1.5	58

Woodson Elevator (304 SS)
  Johnson and Johnson
    Professional, Inc.
  Raynham, MA
	No	1.5	63

References

1. New PFJ, Rosen BR, Brady TJ, et al. Potential hazards and artifacts of ferromagnetic and nonferromagnetic surgical and dental materials and devices in nuclear magnetic resonance imaging. *Radiology* 1983;147:139–148.
2. Becker RL, Norfray JF, Teitelbaum GP, et al. MR imaging in patients with intracranial aneurysm clips. *AJR* 1988;9:885–889.
3. Shellock FG, Crues JV. High-field strength MR imaging and metallic biomedical implants: an ex vivo evaluation of deflection forces. *AJR* 1988;151:389–392.
4. Brown MA, Carden JA, Coleman RE, et al. Magnetic field effects on surgical ligation clips. *Magn Res Imag* 1987;5:443–453.
5. Dujovny M, Kossovsky N, Kossowsky R, et al. Aneurysm clip motion during magnetic resonance imaging: in vivo experimental study with metallurgical factor analysis. *Neurosurgery* 1985;17:543–548.
6. Barrafato D, Henkelman RM. Magnetic resonance imaging and surgical clips. *Can J Surg* 1984;27:509–512.
7. Moscatel M, Shellock FG, Morisoli S. Biopsy needles and devices: assessment of ferromagnetism and artifacts during exposure to a 1.5 Tesla MR system. *J Magn Res Imag* 1995;5:369–372.
8. Shellock FG, Shellock VJ. Additional information pertaining to the MR-compatibility of biopsy needles and devices. *J Magn Res Imag* 1996;6:441.
9. Hathout G, Lufkin RB, Jabour B, et al. MR-guided aspiration cytology in the head and neck at high field strength. *J Magn Res Imag* 1992;2:93–94.
10. Fagan LL, Shellock FG, Brenner RJ, Rothman B. Ex vivo evaluation of ferromagnetism, heating, and artifacts of breast tissue expanders exposed to a 1.5 T MR system. *J Magn Res Imag* 1995;5:614–616.
11. Teitelbaum GP, Lin MCW, Watanabe AT, et al. Ferromagnetism and MR imaging: safety of cartoid vascular clamps. *AJNR* 1990;11:267–272.
12. Gegauff A, Laurell KA, Thavendrarajah A, et al. A potential MRI hazard: forces on dental magnet keepers. *J Oral Rehabil* 1990;17:403–410.

References

13. Shellock FG. Ex vivo assessment of deflection forces and artifacts associated with high-field strength MRI of "mini-magnet" dental prostheses. *Magn Res Imag* 1989;7(suppl 1):38.
14. Shellock FG, Slimp G. Halo vest for cervical spine fixation during MR imaging. *AJR* 1990;154:631–632.
15. Clayman DA, Murakami ME, Vines FS. Compatibility of cervical spine braces with MR imaging. A study of nine nonferrous devices. *AJNR* 1990;11:385–390.
16. Shellock FG. MR imaging and cervical fixation devices: assessment of ferromagnetism, heating, and artifacts. *Magn Res Imag* 1996;14:1093–1098.
17. Soulen RL, Budinger TF, Higgins CB. Magnetic resonance imaging of prosthetic heart valves. *Radiology* 1985;154:705–707.
18. Shellock FG, Morisoli SM. Ex vivo evaluation of ferromagnetism, heating, and artifacts for heart valve prostheses exposed to a 1.5 Tesla MR system. *J Magn Res Imag* 1994;4:756–758.
19. Hassler M, Le Bas JF, Wolf JE, et al. Effects of magnetic fields used in MRI on 15 prosthetic heart valves. *J Radiol* 1986;67:661–666.
20. Frank H, Buxbaum P, Huber L, et al. In vitro behavior of mechanical heart valves in 1.5 T superconducting magnet. *Eur J Radiol* 1992;2:555–558.
21. Teitelbaum GP, Bradley WG, Klein BD. MR imaging artifacts, ferromagnetism, and magnetic torque of intravascular filters, stents, and coils. *Radiology* 1988;166:657–664.
22. Marshall MW, Teitelbaum GP, Kim HS, et al. Ferromagnetism and magnetic resonance artifacts of platinum embolization microcoils. *Cardiovasc Intervent Radiol* 1991;14:163–166.
23. Watanabe AT, Teitelbaum GP, Gomes AS, et al. MR imaging of the bird's nest filter. *Radiology* 1990;177:578–579.
24. Leibman CE, Messersmith RN, Levin DN, et al. MR imaging of inferior vena caval filter: safety and artifacts. *AJR* 1988;150:1174–1176.
25. Shellock FG, Detrick MS, Brant-Zawadski M. MR-compatibility of the Guglielmi detachable coils. *Radiology* 1997;203:568–570.
26. Kiproff PM, Deeb DL, Contractor FM, Khoury MB. Magnetic resonance characteristics of the LGM vena cava filter: technical note. *Cardiovasc Intervent Radiol* 1991;14:254–255.
27. Teitelbaum GP, Raney M, Carvlin MJ, et al. Evaluation of ferromagnetism and magnetic resonance imaging artifacts of the Strecker tantalum vascular stent. *Cardiovasc Intervent Radiol* 1989;12:125–127.

28. Girard MJ, Hahn P, Saini S, Dawson SL, Goldberg MA, Mueller PR. Wallstent metallic biliary endoprosthesis: MR imaging characteristics. *Radiology* 1992;184:874–876.
29. Shellock FG, Myers SM, Schatz CJ. Ex vivo evaluation of ferromagnetism determined for metallic scleral "buckles" exposed to a 1.5 T MR scanner. *Radiology* 1992;185:288–289.
30. de Keizer RJ, Te Strake L. Intraocular lens implants (pseudophakoi) and steelwire sutures: a contraindication for MRI? *Doc Ophthalmol* 1984;61:281–284.
31. Albert DW, Olson KR, Parel JM, et al. Magnetic resonance imaging and retinal tacks. *Arch Ophthalmol* 1990;108:320–321.
32. Joondeph BC, Peyman GA, Mafee MF, et al. Magnetic resonance imaging and retinal tacks [Letter]. *Arch Ophthalmol* 1987;105:1479–1480.
33. Lyons CJ, Betz RR, Mesgarzadeh M, et al. The effect of magnetic resonance imaging on metal spine implants. *Spine* 1989;14:670–672.
34. Shellock FG, Mink JH, Curtin S, et al. MRI and orthopedic implants used for anterior cruciate ligament reconstruction: assessment of ferromagnetism and artifacts. *J Magn Res Imag* 1992;2:225–228.
35. Shellock FG, Schatz CJ. High-field strength MR imaging and metallic otologic implants. *AJNR* 1991;12:279–281.
36. Nogueira M, Shellock FG. Otologic bioimplants: ex vivo assessment of ferromagnetism and artifacts at 1.5 Tesla. *AJR* 1995;163:1472–1473.
37. Mattucci KF, Setzen M, Hyman R, et al. The effect of nuclear magnetic resonance imaging on metallic middle ear prostheses. *Otolaryngol Head Neck Surg* 1986;94:441–443.
38. Applebaum EL, Valvassori GE. Further studies on the effects of magnetic resonance fields on middle ear implants. *Ann Otol Rhinol Laryngol* 1990;99:801–804.
39. White DW. Interaction between magnetic fields and metallic ossicular prostheses. *Am J Otol* 1987;8:290–292.
40. Leon JA, Gabriele OF. Middle ear prosthesis: significance in magnetic resonance imaging. *Magn Reson Imaging* 1987;5:405–406.
41. Shellock FG, Morisoli SM. Ex vivo evaluation of ferromagnetism and artifacts for cardiac occluders exposed to a 1.5 Tesla MR system. *J Magn Res Imag* 1994;4:213–215.
42. Teitelbaum GP, Yee CA, Van Horn DD, et al. Metallic ballistic fragments: MR imaging safety and artifacts. *Radiology* 1990;175:855–859.

43. Shellock FG, Crues JV, Sacks SA. High-field magnetic resonance imaging of penile prostheses: in vitro evaluation of deflection forces and imaging artifacts [Abstract]. In: *Book of Abstracts, Society of Magnetic Resonance in Medicine*. Berkeley, CA: Society of Magnetic Resonance in Medicine;1987;3:915.
44. Shellock FG, Nogueira M, Morisoli S. MR imaging and vascular access ports: ex vivo evaluation of ferromagnetism, heating, and artifacts at 1.5 T. *J Magn Res Imag* 1995;5:481–484.
45. Shellock FG, Shellock VJ. Vascular access ports and catheters tested for ferromagnetism, heating, and artifacts associated with MR imaging. *Magn Reson Imaging* 1996;14:443–447.
46. Kanal E, Shaibani A. Firearm safety in the MR imaging environment. *Radiology* 1994;193:875–876.
47. Hess T, Stepanow B, Knopp MV. Safety of intrauterine contraceptive devices during MR imaging. *Eur Radiol* 1996;6:66–68.
48. Shellock FG, Shellock VJ. Evaluation of MR compatibility of 38 bioimplants and devices. *Radiology* 1995;197:174.
49. Shellock FG, Shellock VJ. Ceramic surgical instruments: ex vivo evaluation of compatibility with MR imaging. *J Magn Res Imag* 1996;6:954–956.
50. Shellock FG, Shellock VJ. Evaluation of cranial flap fixation clamps for compatibility with MR imaging. *Radiology* 1998;822–825.
51. Lufkin R, Jordan S, Lylcyk M. MR imaging with topographic EEG electrodes in place. *AJNR* 1988;9:953–954.
52. Marra S, Leonetti JP, Konior RJ, Raslan W. Effect of magnetic resonance imaging on implantable eyelid weights. *Ann Otol Rhinol Laryngol* 1995;104:448–452.
53. Zhang J, Wilson CL, Levesque MF, et al. Temperature changes in nickel-chromium intracranial depth electrodes during MR scanning. *AJNR* 1993;14:497–500.
54. Mark AS, Hricak H. Intrauterine contraceptive devices: MR imaging. *Radiology* 1987;162:311–314.
55. Go KG, Kamman RL, Mooyaart EL. Interaction of metallic neurosurgical implants with magnetic resonance imaging at 1.5 Tesla as a cause of image distortion and of hazardous movement of the implant. *Clin Neurosurg* 1989;91:109–115.
56. Fransen P, Dooms G, Thauvoy R. Safety of the adjustable pressure ventricular valve in magnetic resonance imaging: problems and solutions. *Neuroradiology* 1992;34:508–509.
57. ECRI, Health devices alert. A new MRI complication? May 27, 1988.

58. To SYC, Lufkin RB, Chiu L. MR-compatible winged infusion set. *Comput Med Imag Graph* 1989;13:469–472.
59. Shellock FG, Shellock VJ. MR-compatibility evaluation of the Spetzler titanium aneurysm clip. *Radiology* 1998;206:838–841.
60. Shellock FG. MR-compatibility of an endoscope designed for use in interventional MRI procedures. *AJR* 1998;71:1297–1300.
61. Shellock FG, Shellock VJ. Cardiovascular catheters and accessories: ex vivo testing of ferromagnetism, heating, and artifacts associated with MRI. *J Magn Res Imag* 1998;8:1338–1342.
62. Shellock FG, Shellock VJ. Metallic marking clips used after stereotactic breast biopsy: ex vivo testing of ferromagnetism, heating, and artifacts associated with MRI. *AJR* (all in press).
63. Shellock FG. MRI safety of instruments designed for interventional MRI: assessment of ferromagnetism, heating, and artifacts. *Workshop on New Insights into Safety and Compatibility Issues Affecting In Vivo MR, Syllabus,* 1998;pp. 39.
64. Shellock FG, Hatfield M, Simon BJ, et al. Implantable spinal fusion stimulator: assessment of MRI safety. *AJR* (in press).
65. Shellock FG, Shellock VJ. Stents: Evaluation of MRI safety. *AJR* (in press).
66. Teissl C, Kremser C, Hochmair ES, Hochmair Desoyer IJ. Cochlear implants: in vitro investigation of electromagnetic interference at MR imaging-compatibility and safety aspects. *Radiology* 1998;208:700–708.
67. Teissl C, Kremser C, Hochmair ES, Hochmair-Desoyer IJ. Magnetic resonance imaging and cochlear implants: compatibility and safety aspects. *J Magn Res Imag* 1999;9:26–38.
68. Ortler M, Kostron H, Felber S. Transcutaneous pressure-adjustable valves and magnetic resonance imaging: an ex vivo examination of the Codman-Medos programmable valve and the Sophy adjustable pressure valve. *Neurosurgery* 1997;40:1050–1057.

Appendix I
Medical Devices Developed for Interventional MR Procedures*

Various vendors, prompted by the recommendations and requests from MR users, have recognized the need for developing specialized medical devices, equipment, and instruments necessary to facilitate the performance of interventional MRI procedures. Similar to other devices utilized in the MR environment, *ex vivo* testing and evaluation is required to demonstrate the safe use and operation of these instruments and devices before utilization in interventional MR procedures. The test procedures include an assessment of magnetic field attraction, heating, induced current (for certain devices) and artifacts using standardized techniques. Medical devices can then be characterized with respect to being "MR-compatible," "MR-safe," or "MR-tested," with the electromagnetic fields of the MR environment. This appendix provides a comprehensive listing of vendors who are a source for a variety of devices, instruments, and equipment that were designed for interventional MRI procedures. Information is indicated regarding the specific products that each vendor makes as well as a person to contact who specializes in this unique product line.

AESCULAP, INC.
1000 Gateway Blvd.
So. San Francisco, CA 94080
Product(s)
General Surgical Instruments
Catalog or Special Items
MR safe surgical instruments
Contact:
Haio F. Fauser
New Business Development Manager, U.S.
Phone: 800-282-9000 or 415-876-7000
International Contact
Paul Wieneke (1st contact)
Phone: 49-74-61-95-2801; Fax: 49-74-61-146-14
Aesculap AG
AM Aesculap-Platz
P.O. Box 40
78501 Tuttlingen/Germany

BIP
AM Brand 1
P.C. 0-82299 Tuerkenfeld, Germany
Product(s)
Core biopsy gun
Contact
Norbert Hece
Phone: 49-81936026 or 49-81936548
International Contact
Same

COGENT LIGHT
26145 Technology Drive
Santa Clarita, CA 91355-1137
Product(s)
Headlight/Lightsource
Contact
Richard B. Davies
Phone: 805-294-2989; Fax: 805-294-2904 (800-294-2989 #101)

Appendix I

COOK MEDICAL
P.O. Box 489
Bloomington, IN 47402
Product(s)
Needles, biopsy guns, catheters
Contact
John DeFord, Ph.D.
Product Development Manager
Phone: 812-339-2235; Fax: 812-339-5369
Toll-Free: 800-346-2686
Customer Service: 800-457-4500
International Contact
Same

CRYOMEDICAL SCIENCES
1300 Piccard Drive, Suite 102
Rockville, MD 20850
Product(s)
Cryotherapy equipment
Contact
John Baust
Vice President of Research & Development
Phone: 301-417-7070; Fax: 301-417-7077
International Contact
German Distributor:
Uwe Lindmfller
B&K Medical
Phone: 49-5143-93227; Fax: 49-5143-93228

CUDA PRODUCTS
600 Powers Avenue
Jacksonville, FL 32217
Product(s)
Adaptors for light source to the endoscope
Catalog or Special Items
Olympus C-0200
Wolff C-0201
ACMI C-0202
Contact
Phone: 904-737-7611; Fax: 904-733-4832

DAUM CORPORATION
UMBC Technology Center
1450 South Rolling Road
Baltimore, MD 21227

Product(s)
Needles

Contact
Phone: 410-455-5786; Fax: 410-455-5787
Email: info@cadaum.de or medinfo@cadaum.de

International Contact
Daum GmbH Deutschland
Wolfgang Daum, President
Hagenower Strasse 73
D-19061 Schwerin
Phone: 49-385-6344-344; Fax: 49-385-6344-152

DORNIER MEDIZINLASER GMBH
Industriestrasse 15
82110 Germering, Germany

Products
MR-safe laser-delivery-systems and
various MR-safe applicators
for laser induced-thermotherapy (LITT)

Contact
Wolfgang Illich
Development Engineer
Phone: 49-89-84108-133; Fax: 49-89-84108-745
Email: wolfgang.illich@cadomedtech.de
Dr. Werner Rother
Sales Manager
Phone: 49-89-84108-640; Fax: 49-89-84108-552
Email: werner.rother@cadomedtech.de

E-Z-EM, INC
717 Main Street
Westbury, NY 11590

Product(s)
Lufkin 22 gauge cytology biopsy needles
MRI histology biopsy needles

Appendix I

MRI core biopsy guns, 14 and 18 gauge
MRI lesion marking systems (20 gauge needle with Kopans style localization wire)
Electrosurgical instruments

Direct Sale or Distribution
Both, but primarily through distributors on six continents

Contact
Andy Zwarun, Vice President
Phone: 516-333-8230, ext. 304; Fax: 516-333-8278
Email: anzwar@caworldnet.att.net

International Contact
Germany: Edwin Schneider (Guerbet)
Phone: 49-6196-7620; Fax: 49-6196-79934
Switzerland: Christopher Jackson
Manager, Medilink
Phone: 41-91-972-8417; Fax: 41-91-972-8568

ERBE ELEKTROMEDIZIN GMBH

Waldhoernlestrasse 17
72072 Tuebingen, Germany
General Phone number: 49-7071-755-0
ERBE USA Inc.
2225 Northwest Parkway, Suite 105
Marietta, GA 30067

Product(s)
Electrosurgical Equipment: ICC 350-MRI
(MR-safe generator allowing mono- and bipolar operation), instruments and accessories
Cryosurgery units

Contact
Germany:
Martin Hagg
VP Design & Engineering
Phone: 49-7071-755-249; Fax: 49-7071-755-549
Email: mhagg@caerbe-med.de
U.S.A.:
David Hartnett
Vice President, Marketing
Phone: 800-778-3723; Fax: 770-955-2577

GROUPE BRUKER ODAM
34, rue de l'industrie
Wissembourg, France 67160
Product(s)
Patient monitoring
Contact
Laurent Sigrist
Secretaire General
Phone: 33-88-63-36-06; Fax: 33-88-54-36-32
Sales Department:
Phone: 33-88-63-36-00; Fax: 33-88-94-12-82
International Contact
Same as above

INTERMETRO INDUSTRIES
North Washington Street
Wilkes-Barre, PA 17805
Product(s)
Drug/storage carts
Contact
Phone: 717-825-2741; Fax: 717-825-2852
E-mail: imet@cavds.net

ITI MEDICAL TECHNOLOGIES
2452 Armstrong Street
Livermore, CA 94550
Product(s)
"Prototype" devices, Biopsy Needle
Contact
Roger W. Werne, Ph.D.
Phone: 510-371-8305; Fax: 510-371-8222

IN-VIVO RESEARCH
4420 Metric Drive, Suite A
Winter Park, FL 32792
Product(s)
Vital sign monitoring equipment capable of monitoring ECG, respiratory, invasive and noninvasive blood pressure, and temperature

Catalog or Special Items
  All products have been 510K cleared for MRI use and are standard catalog items
Direct Sale or Distribution
  Market through direct sales reps with some distributors
Contact
  Christopher Dedyo
  Director of Marketing
  Phone: 407-275-3220; Fax: 407-249-2022
International Contact
  Sally Dugan
  International Sales Manager
  Orlando Office

J&J ETHICON, INC.
  Route 22
  Somerville, NJ 08876
Product(s)
  Needles with sutures
Contact
  Bill McJames
  Phone: 908-218-2297; Fax: 908-218-2531

JOHNSON & JOHNSON PROFESSIONAL, INC. (CODMAN DIVISION)
  41 Pacella Park Drive
  Randolph, MA 02368
Product(s)
  CMC3 Irrigation Bi-polar, Bookwalter Arm and Table Post, Rhoton
  Microsurgical, Hudson Twist Drill
Direct Sale or Distribution
  Direct sales through representatives
Contact
  Paula Papineau
  Associate Product Director
  Greg Auda
  Director of Instrumentation
  Phone: 508-828-3228; Fax: 508-828-3065

Appendix I

International Contact
  Blair Fraser
  Manager of new business development for
  European operation
  Phone: 44-13 44-86 40 30

LIFE INSTRUMENTS
  14 Wood Road
  Braintree, MA 02184
Product(s)
  Penfields, Curettes, Mini Cobbs, Hudson
  Twist Drill, Drill Bits, Periosteal
  Elevators
Contact
  Larry Foley
  Phone: 617-849-0209 or 800-925-2995
  Fax: 617-849-0128
International Contact
  Same

LONE PEAK ENGINEERING
  12660 S. Fort Street
  Draper, Utah 84020
Product(s)
  Ceramic Scissors C-124
Contact
  Vickey Coombes
  Phone: 801-553-1732; Fax: 801-553-1734
International Contact
  Same as above, initially

MAGNETIC RESONANCE EQUIPMENT CORPORATION
  P.O. Box 5489
  5 Grant Avenue
  Bay Shore, NY 11706
Product(s)
  Patient monitors and patient communication and music systems
Catalog or Special Items
  Catalog

Direct Sale or Distribution
  Direct in the U.S. and Canada and through dealers in the rest of the world
Contact
  John V. Plump
  Phone: 516-243-3500; Fax: 516-243-3516

MAGNETIC VisiOn GMBH
  Lochacher 6
  CH-8630 Ruti, Switzerland
Product(s)
  Neurosurgery Drill, Neurobiopsy Needle Guide, Dura hook, Retractor
International Contact
  Dr. Adriano Vigano
  Phone: 41-55-260-1855; Fax: 41-55-260-1859
  E-mail: A Vigano@caswissonline.ch

MEDILAS AG
  Grindlenstrasse 3
  CH-8954 Geroldswil, Switzerland
Product(s)
  Drapes
Direct Sale or Distribution
  Distributor
International Contact
  Mark Kleger
  Phone: 41-1-748-4000; Fax: 41-1-748-0105

MEDRAD
  240 Alpha Drive
  Pittsburgh, PA 15238-2870
Product(s)
  Spectris MR Injector
  (For injection of contrast media only, and explicitly not for drug or chemotherapy infusion.)
Contact
  Phone: 800-633-7237 or 412-967-9700
  Fax: 412-963-1964

International Contact
  Medrad Europe
  Postbus 3084
  NL-6202 N.B. Maastricht, The Netherlands
  Phone: 31-43-364-08-08; Fax: 31-43-365-00-20
  Brigette Paltra (Meditron)
  Phone: 41-55-4502121; Fax: 41-62-3900315

MIDAS REX, L.P.
  3001 Race Street
  Ft. Worth, TX 76111
Product(s)
  Pneumatic drill
Contact
  Gary B. Gage
  Director of R&D
  Phone: 817-831-2604 or 800-433-7639
  Fax: 817-834-4835

MÖLLER MICROSURGICAL
  7 Industrial Park
  Waldwick, NJ 07463
Product(s)
  Microscope
Contact
  Dick Montgomery
  Vice President, Marketing & Sales
  Phone: 201-251-9592; Fax: 201-251-9516
International Contact
  Dr. Martin Schmidt, President
  J.D. Möller Optische Werke GmbH
  Rosengarten 10
  D-22880 Wedel/Germany
  Phone: 04103-70-93-33; Fax: 04103-70-93-50

MR RESOURCES, INC.
  158R Main Street, P.O. Box 880
  Gardner, MA 01440

Product(s)
  MR parts and accessories, stethoscopes
Catalog or Special Items
  Catalog items
Direct Sale or Distribution
  Direct
Contact
  Ann Cochran, Catalog Manager
  Phone: 800-443-5486 or 508-632-7000
International Contact
  Same

NORTH AMERICAN DRAEGER
  3136 Quarry Road
  Telford, PA 18969
Product(s)
  MRI anesthesia unit with electronic ventilator, and monitoring system
Catalog or Special Items
  Catalog
Direct Sale or Distribution
  Direct
Contact
  Greg Sutherland
  Product Manager
  Phone: 800-462-7566

OHMEDA INC.
  Ohmeda Drive, P.O. Box 7550
  Madison, WI 53707-7550
Product(s)
  Anesthesia machines, vaporizers, breathing circuit
Catalog or Special Items
  Catalog items
Direct Sale or Distribution
  Direct
Contact
  Deb Schmaling
  Marketing Product Manager for Excell
  Phone: 800-345-2700, ext. 3357

Fax: 608-223-2476
Email: deb.schmaling@caohmeda.boc.com

OLYMPUS AMERICA
4 Nevada Dr.
Lake Success, NY 11042-1179
Product(s)
Endoscopes, light sources, video systems
Contact
Gene Eldrige
Senior Design Engineer
Research & Development, Medical Instr. Div.
Phone: 516-844-5467; Fax: 516-326-9085

OMI SURGICAL PRODUCTS
3924 Virginia Avenue
Cincinnati, OH 45227
Product(s)
Mayfield Skull Clamp
Catalog or Special Items
MR Safe Skull Pins
Contact
Chuck Dinkler
Research & Development
Phone: 800-755-6381 or 513-561-2705
Fax: 513-561-0195
International Contact
Same

OMNIVENT
1720 Sublette Ave.
St. Louis, MO 63110
Product(s)
Patient ventilation and ventilator monitors
Catalog or Special Items
Both
Direct Sale or Distribution
Both

Appendix I

Contact
  Bill Gates, President
  Phone: 800-933-7902 or 913-273-8924

PACIFIC SURGICAL INNOVATIONS, INC.
  871 Industrial Road, Unit A
  San Carlos, CA 94070
Product(s)
  Neurosurgical Instruments
Catalog or Special Items
  Catalog
Direct Sale or Distribution
Contact
  Terry Johnston
  Phone: 800-810-6610 or 415-802-6988
  Fax: 415-802-0120
International Contact
  U.S. only

PENLON
  Abingdon,
  Oxon, England OX14 3PH
Product(s)
  MR Safe Ventilator
  Nuffield, Series 200
Direct Sale or Distribution
  Available worldwide
Contact
  Craig Thompson
  Marketing Manager
  Phone: 44-1235-554-222; Fax: 44-1235-555-252
International Contact
  Same as above

PFIZER-SCHNEIDER
  P.O. Box+Ackerstrasse 6
  Bflach, Switzerland CH-8180
Product(s)
  Diagnostic catheters with MR tracking tips

Contact
  Eugene Hofmann
  Manager, Research & Development
  Phone: 41-1-872-1111; Fax: 41-1-862-0504
International Contact
  Same as above

PINA-VERTRIEBS AG
  Langrietstr. 17a
  Neuhausen 2/Sh, Switzerland CH-8212
Product(s)
  Surgical instruments, development of MR-safe custom devices, implants, scissors
Catalog or Special Items
  Willing to fabricate MR compatible scissors in any size and shape
International Contact
  Axel Hoehn
  Director of Sales and Marketing
  Phone: 41-52-672-40-42; Fax: 41-52-672-40-48
  Mobile: 49-171-349 41-19

(Deknatel) SNOWDEN PENCER
  5175 S. Royal Atlanta Drive
  Tucker, GA 30084
Product(s)
  Titanium surgical instruments
Catalog or Special Items
  Catalog
Direct Sale or Distribution
  Direct only
Contact
  Customer Service Department
  Phone: 800-367-7874 or 770-934-4922
International Contact
  Snowden-Pencer Customer Service Dept.
  Phone: 770-496-0952

SOMATEX
  Postfach 420620
  D-12066 Berlin, Germany

Product(s)
  MR Compatible Needles
Contact
  Frank Kniep
  Phone: 49-30-625-3046; Fax: 49-30-625-3047
International Contact
  Same

STERILE CONCEPTS
  5100 Commerce Road
  Richmond, VA 23234
Product(s)
  Custom Healthcare Procedure Trays
Catalog or Special Items
  Supplies Brigham & Women's Hospital with their MRI Biopsy Pack (Order #BX9123A)
Contact
  Phone: 804-236-0260; Fax: 804-236-7255

STUDER MEDICAL ENGINEERING
  Rundbuckstraße 2
  CH-8212 Neuhausen am Reinfall, Switzerland
Product(s)
  Moeller Microscopes and Stand
Contact
  Rudolf Hensler
  Phone: 41-52-674-0878; Fax: 41-52-674-0879
  Karl Weissbach
  Mobile: 49-171-210-6812

SWANN-MOTOR LIMITED
  Owlerton Green
  Sheffield, S6 2BJ, England
Product(s)
  Surgical Handles in nickel
Contact
  Phone: 0114-234-4231; Fax: 0114-231-4966

Appendix I

SYNERGETICS, INC
17466 Chesterfield Airport Road
Chesterfield, MO 63005
Product(s)
Deep Neuro Dissection Set
Synerturn N000-160
Contact
Ed Tinn
Phone: 314-530-1440; Fax: 314-530-1143
To order: 800-600-0565

SYNTHES
1690 Russell Road
Paoli, PA 19301
Catalog or Special Items
Maxillo-Facial Plating System
Contact
Paul J. Gordon
Group Product Manager
Phone: 610-647-9700
International Contact
Same

UNITED METAL FABRICATORS
409 Eisenhauer Boulevard
Johnstown, PA 15904
Product(s)
Instrument tables, basin stands, OR furniture, case carts, etc.
Contact
Peter Terry
1-800-638-5322 or 814-266-8726
FAX: 814-266-1870

US SURGICAL
150 Glover Avenue
Norwalk, CT 06856
Product(s)
10 mm Surgiview Scope #176608, accessories

Contact
John Tovey
Phone: 617-533-1017

VALLEY FORGE SCIENTIFIC CORP.
136 Green Tree Road, Suite 100
Oaks, PA 19456
Product(s)
VFS-200 Bi-polar unit, electrocautery
Contact
Jerry Malis, Ph.D.
Bonnie Ritchie
Phone: 610-666-7500; Fax: 610-666-7565
International Contact
Same

VEENSTRA INSTRUMENTS
Madame Curieweg 1
P.O. Box 115
Nl-8500 Ac Joure, The Netherlands
Product(s)
Trolleys, case carts, OR furniture
Contact
Headquarters
Phone: 31-513-41-69-64; Fax: 31-513-41-69-19

*Special thanks to Ms. Karen Streit of General Electric Medical Systems, Milwaukee, WI for providing the majority of the information for this list.

Note that some of the medical devices, equipment, and instruments may be pre-product prototypes that do have completed evaluations by the U.S. Food and Drug Administration (FDA), European CE Mark or other reviews for safety or effectiveness that may be necessary prior to commercial distribution of these devices. Some devices may not be available in all countries. No claims are made regarding patient/staff safety, MR compatibility, MR safety, or clinical capability of any of the medical devices included in this list. Before introduction of any medical device into the MRI suite, the device should be inspected by qualified hospital personnel. The non-magnetic properties of the device and its clinical operation in the magnetic field should be verified before it is used in an interventional MR procedure. Use of these medical devices for animal or human procedures must comply with any applicable government or local hospital safety and animal/human studies committee requirements. Interventional MRI sites should contact the vendors directly for technical specifications, pricing and commercial availability of the medical products.

Appendix II

Email Address for Frank G. Shellock, Ph.D.

If you have a specific question about a bioimplant, material, or device, or testing of a medical product please contact Frank G. Shellock, Ph.D. at: **shellock@flash.net**

Frank G. Shellock, Ph.D. is an Adjunct Clinical Professor of Radiology at University of Southern California and the President of Shellock R & D Services, Inc. He is a Member of the Safety Committees for the International Society for Magnetic Resonance Imaging and American College of Radiology and a former member of the Board of Directors of the Society for Magnetic Resonance Imaging. Dr. Shellock is a Fellow of the American College of Sportsmedicine and a Reviewing Editor for nine biomedical journals. He has published four textbooks, more than 50 book chapters, and more than 140 peer-reviewed articles. Dr. Shellock's current research interests and endeavors include investigations designed to implement new MR imaging techniques for the musculoskeletal system, to develop new clinical applications for MRI procedures, to evaluate electromagnetic field-related bioeffects, and to develop instruments and devices used for interventional MR procedures. He continues to test and characterize the MRI safety aspects of bioimplants, devices, and materials.

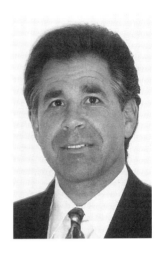